Maximizing Your Energy & Personal Productivity

Maximizing Your Energy & Personal Productivity

Charles T. Kuntzleman Ed.D.

NordicPress

Notice: The information and ideas in this book are for educational purposes and are not intended as prescriptive advice. Consult your physician before starting any exercise or weight loss program.

Library of Congress Catalog Card Number: 91-66984

ISBN: 0-9627708-2-5

Printed in the United States of America

Table of Contents

Introduction

For almost 30 years now I've been trying to help people live well. I've tried to convince them to help themselves to a better life and to then convince others to do the same.

I've also listened carefully to what people say to me. Most people don't talk about improving their health. Instead, they talk about increasing their energy levels, about having more get-up-and-go. One woman told me, "I'm so low on the energy scale that the best part of the day is over when my alarm clock goes off."

Finding a Zest for Living

Energy is your zest for working, playing, loving—living. It is your physical capacity for living and your mental attitude toward your capacity for living. In practical terms, you have "energy" if you can get through your working day with enough physical resources to meet unexpected demands, and still enjoy life.

We all know when we have energy. We have felt its rush when taking a walk in the crisp, fall air; upon receiving a hard-earned promotion or raise; anticipating Christmas morning; or reacting to a dangerous situation such as a near car accident. With the rush we become acutely alert, vibrant, and quick-thinking. Life is exciting. Sleep or drowsiness has no place.

We also know when we don't have energy: the drowsiness after a big meal; the fatigue after hours of Christmas shopping; the unresponsiveness we feel on a hot, humid afternoon. We understand such fatigue. What really concerns us is the burn-out some of us feel. We enter employment full of great enthusiasm and vigor, but before the task is completed we notice that our drive and desire have waned.

The Secrets of More Energy

Why do some people have more energy than others? To find the answer I became an observer of human nature. The more I observed, the more it became apparent that energetic people have certain common characteristics. Also, while energy levels vary from person to person, the true energizers are maximizing their energy potentials.

Their characteristics? Energizing people tend to be more fit, eat better foods, are relatively slim, enjoy life, handle change well, get along well with their counterparts, and have a strong sense of control and direction in their lives. They understand that it is their individual responsibility to improve their energy levels and not to depend on external sources such as cigarettes, alcohol, drugs, or excessive caffeine.

You probably know some high-energy people, full of vigor, drive, and a love for living. You'll find that they have many of the characteristics I've mentioned. Such people will tell you there aren't any pat answers to maximum personal energy. I agree. But there are steps that you can take to improve your energy level. And that's what this book is all about. Although the guidelines I have provided are simple, following them is not. But it can be done with less effort than you might think. And I am confident you will find the results energizing.

▶▶▶▶▶▶ Section I: ▶▶▶

The American Way

Change: Prelude to Stress

Years ago, the roof of the Kemper Arena in Kansas City collapsed. Fortunately, the 7,000-ton concrete and steel cover came down when the building was unoccupied, so no one was injured. While the dust was still settling a special team of "structural detectives" arrived on the scene and began climbing around the rubble. Some three months after the mishap the team had analyzed the data and announced the cause of the spectacular accident: stress. One giant steel bolt, responsible for connecting two massive girders, had broken under stress.

So Much to Do, So Little Time

It doesn't take a team of detectives to discover the same thing is happening to a majority of North American people. Surveys indicate that 70 to 90 percent of us are plagued by high levels of stress. To most of us the "rat race" is no longer a joke, but a frightful reality, as we try to cram 25 hours of activity into an already cramped 24-hour day.

The rapid rate at which our society experiences change is one of the primary reasons why our levels of stress are so high. Things are moving so fast that we just can't keep up with them. And there's no getting around it. In today's world, you simply cannot escape change. We are in the midst of what Alvin Toffler calls "future shock." Future shock occurs because you are unsure; unsure about what will happen tomorrow, next year, or in the next decade. You can't be sure because you're right in the midst of rapid change.

Surprisingly, even pleasant changes can produce levels of stress that can be immobilizing. Working with 5,000 patients in a special project, researchers from the University of Washington School of Medicine found that changes in an individual's lifestyle were often accompanied by changes in health. Although negative life changes such as the death of a spouse, divorce, or imprisonment have the biggest impact, even desirable changes such as marriage, retirement, or an outstanding personal achievement may create stress. These clusters of life changes are cumulative, and gradually build up to a "life crisis." Such a crisis can lower your energy levels and make you feel utterly washed out, too tired to do a thing.

In order to survive, people must continually adapt to change. It's pervasive and inescapable, which, of course, means that the accompanying stress is impossible to avoid. In fact, efforts to avoid stress often produce more stress.

According to the late Dr. Hans Selye, the world's leading authority on stress, the absence of stress is death. I know that statement seems strange, but what he's really saying is that stress is essential for life. What is necessary is a balance, and an understanding that stress should be changed to a positive rather than a negative force.

The usual approach to a problem is to try to eliminate it. But stress cannot and should not be eliminated from your life. It can be the spice of life. So what do you do? Develop a grin-and-bear-it attitude? Hold on and hope for the best? A far better solution is to learn how best to cope with it.

Turning Stress into Energy

In reality, stress is simply something of a neutral element. It is neither good nor bad in itself. What makes stress good or bad is how we handle it. Perhaps two examples might help explain this.

I have a friend who is a salesman. By any standard, his world is filled with pressure. The month-end tally is the biggest indicator of whether he has made it or not. Even Jack's play is competitive. Put him on a golf course and he plays like Arnold Palmer. Get him on a handball court and he's a tiger. He works hard and plays hard. He loves his wife and three kids. He spends time during the week and weekends with them. Jack loves it. He's always on top of things, never sick. A real "energy" type of guy.

On most stress inventories, he would score in the "highly stressed" category. You would suspect such things as fatigue, high blood pressure, perhaps an alcohol problem, ulcers, and heart trouble. Instead, Jack has an unbelievable amount of energy and stamina. Why? For Jack, the challenge of making it as a salesman is just the ingredient that makes life exciting and worthwhile. He made it his spice of life. He successfully turned stress into a positive element.

Now take Norman. Norman had inherited a family business that was an established firm. When he took over he added a subsidiary that allowed him to do his own thing—remodeling. In time, he sold the family business for a good profit and retained his small remodeling company.

Today, his working conditions are ideal. He doesn't have to go to work if he doesn't want to. He doesn't have to worry about his income. His home is very comfortable and well appointed. He tells me that he and his wife have a good relationship. His two children are doing well in school. His home is paid for and he's bought a vacation spot on Lake Michigan. He will soon celebrate his twentieth wedding anniversary. He flies his own plane and travels extensively. In short, Norman seems to have it made.

Surprisingly, Norman is a very unhappy man. Despite the fact that he apparently experiences little stress, he complains of chronic fatigue. He has all of the symptoms of high-level stress, yet most stress inventories score him in the "mellow" range. Norman's orderly and calm life is causing the stress. The very lack of change has become a stressful point with him. He's frustrated, hostile, and angry. He wants to do something to prove himself, but he's afraid; afraid that he'll fail financially and his secure environment will be shattered.

Of course, these stories aren't typical, but they illustrate a very important point. The level of stress and change is not what differentiates these people; it's their attitude. Jack doesn't have fatigue or lack of energy. He enjoys what he's doing and is coping very well. Norman has troubles—he's coping improperly. Norman has let stress become *distress.* And that's where energy enters the picture.

The Relationship of Stress to Energy

Since we cannot avoid stress, we have two responses available to us. We can be governed by stress and allow it to destroy us, or we can meet it efficiently and enjoy it. The first response depletes our supply of energy, the second adds to it. It's almost that simple.

In the 1930's, Selye coined a phrase to describe how stress affects the human body. He called it "the general adaptation syndrome," comprising three responses to stress: alarm, resistance, and exhaustion. The alarm stage is the sense of excitement you get when the boss calls at 7:00 a.m. and asks you to come to work early. You get a surge of adrenaline that increases your pulse rate and, perhaps, some perspiration under your arms. Blood pressure rises, muscles tense. You're hyped up and ready to go. This response is rather short and often is good for you. For example, if you heard the smoke alarm in the middle of the night, the extra dose of adrenaline your body receives may allow you to perform superhuman efforts to get your family to safety. In this stage, stress produces energy to help you complete a task.

If the stress continues, the alarm stage changes to resistance. That is, rather than reacting, your body has decided to fight. The pituitary gland produces hormones that equip your body for a longer contest. One hormone, vasopressin, raises your blood pressure, while another, thyrotrophic hormone (TSH), stimulates your thyroid gland, thus accelerating your metabolism. Still another hormone, called adrenocorticotrophic hormone (ACTH), elevates blood sugar levels and alters your immune system. All of these changes provide the sustained energy necessary to keep going.

Under normal circumstances, the second stage gives way to exhaustion, and the body is allowed to rest and recover. This could be characterized by a singularly rough day at the office. You were still in the alarm stage when you got to your desk and found a note from the boss telling you to have a difficult report to him by 3:00 p.m. The initial boost of adrenaline gave you the drive to get right at it. Soon you were busy trying to make the deadline despite numerous phone interruptions. Things went quite well because the resistance phase was providing your system with the necessary stimulus to meet the challenge. When you got home, you were able to relax, read the newspaper, enjoy a nice meal, and go to bed early.

If everyone followed that pattern of adaptation to stress, there would be no need for advice on stress. However, when the stress continues without an exhaustion phase, it becomes a very real energy-related problem. Stress at the office, insufficient finances, deteriorating relationships, and nagging doubts about self-worth result in this crippling cycle: stress, mental exhaustion, more stress, insomnia, chronic fatigue, more stress, etc.

Finding a Healthy Balance

Inborn traits play a crucial role in stress. For example, Selye says some people are born to be race horses and others to be turtles. Forcing a race horse to be a turtle, and vice versa, creates significant stress. This is the mistake of the Type A and Type B advocates.

Drs. Mayer Friedman and Ray Rosemann from San Francisco have postulated that certain people are more prone to coronary disease: Type A personalities try to squeeze 25 hours in 24; take on more and more responsibilities with less and less time; try to do two or more things at a time (such as shaving and driving a car); have a difficult time saying no; are very punctual and competitive; and do not take time to enjoy their environment. They are the classic workaholics.

At the other end of the spectrum are the Type B's, who take a more relaxed approach to life. They are productive, but they tackle one task at a time, are less impatient, accept themselves, and take time to stop and smell the roses. Rosemann and Friedman advocate that a Type A should adopt more of Type B's behavior characteristics.

Quite frankly, I have problems with the Type A/Type B concept as it is usually presented. First, I find it ludicrous to classify five billion people into two distinct categories, A or B. Second, trying to change a supposedly Type A person into a Type B person is stress-producing. If a person likes himself or herself as he or she is, there is no reason to change.

Third, the real issue is not Type A versus Type B. It's the traits that Rosemann and Friedman tacked on at the end of their definition—that Type A people are angry, hostile, impatient, aggressive, and that they view life as a struggle. If you have those behavior characteristics, you're in trouble, whether you're Type A or Type B. You're not coping well with your environment. However, I know people who are happy, outgoing, productive, and fun-loving, yet they have Type A personalities. Many Type B people are the same way, but I also know some B's who are very angry, competitive, hostile, and impatient. Life to them is a struggle.

Some stress-management people might argue with me, but I feel the emphasis should be on the devastating attitudes and behaviors associated with anger, impatience, and struggle. These characteristics are an indication that the affected individuals are not coping very well with stress or change in their environment.

Stress need not rob you of energy. The key to stress and energy is how you handle it—whether you can manage stress or allow it to manage you. You must remember that stress can be the very element that makes life exciting. It would be impossible to enjoy sex, love, a football game, a breath of fresh air, a good book, or music without your hormones that respond to stress. While stress can be debilitating it can also add a tremendous zest to your life. You must find the proper balance.

Fellowship of the Fatigued

The very word fatigue makes me tired. I would just as soon not mention it at all. But you can't talk about energy without dealing with the problem of fatigue. While it is true that our energy level potentials are dictated by heredity, it is apparent that many people are not reaching their optimum level of performance. Fatigue, for whatever reason, is short-circuiting their maximum personal energy.

Fatigue: What Is It?

Fatigue means different things to different people. First, there are two kinds of fatigue: acute and chronic. Acute fatigue is easy to identify. A carpenter, after swinging a hammer for eight hours, would think something was wrong if his arm wasn't fatigued. Run a marathon sometime and see if that doesn't leave you bushed. These are examples of acute fatigue. The cure is simple: a little rest and relaxation.

In this book I'm not concerned about this type of fatigue. It is easily recognized and readily cured. Furthermore, acute fatigue represents no long-term drain on your personal energy reserves. In fact, I view acute fatigue as a good symptom, evidence that you are already performing at high energy levels, needing only occasional recuperation breaks.

The other type of fatigue—chronic fatigue—concerns me. Those who suffer from chronic fatigue don't get tired once in a while. They stay tired, week after week, month after month, year after year. The fatigue does not lessen with rest, recreation, or medication. And, occasionally, when it does subside it returns in a matter of days or weeks.

A thorough physical examination by a physician often reveals nothing. But the patient complains, "I don't have the energy I once had. Things are a drag." These feelings are real. It's been estimated that half the people who see their family physician have nothing organically wrong with them, just overwhelming fatigue or a feeling that they lack energy.

Chronic fatigue, simply stated, is a pervasive feeling of a total shortage of energy. If you're able to function at all, it is only due to an immense effort of the will. You feel as though the force of gravity has doubled when it comes to getting out of bed in the morning. Relationships seem to require more effort than they're worth. Your job is like a dead weight. You wonder why you've stayed with it so long. Your very shoes seem to have rubber cement gumming up their soles, holding you back. A tremendous amount of willpower must be mustered to do anything out of the daily routine of things. And even the daily routine can get to be too much. How many times have you thought, "I'm too tired to get off the couch and crawl into bed"? That's chronic fatigue.

People who suffer from this type of chronic fatigue are from all socioeconomic classes. They include corporate ladder climbers, decision makers, custodians, teachers, ministers, housewives, truck drivers, doctors, students, and so forth. They find themselves physically and emotionally bankrupt. Their brain seems to have wilted and all body functions have gone limp with it.

Scientists tell us there are three types of chronic fatigue: physical, mental, and emotional. These three are so closely intertwined that it is impossible to separate them. But to help you better understand them, I'm separating them here so you can see their influence on your energy levels. Remember, though, that they are closely related. Physical fatigue can cause emotional fatigue, emotional fatigue can cause mental fatigue, and mental fatigue can drain you both physically and emotionally.

Physical Fatigue

Physical fatigue may have physiological or pathological causes. Your level of physical fitness dictates when your daily physical fatigue will occur and how long you will be able to hold it off. For example, a fit person may be able to do his daily chores and then go out for an evening of partying, dancing, or socializing. The unfit person, on the other hand, may be exhausted by two or three o'clock in the afternoon, and find taking a walk in the evening impossible.

Pathological fatigue, on the other hand, includes fatigue due to high blood pressure, diabetes, obesity, hypoglycemia, and arteriosclerosis. In other words, fatigue caused by some disease. I have a good friend, Dave, who suffers from high blood pressure that is hereditary. He is whipped by four o'clock in the afternoon. When he wakes up he feels good, but as the day wears on his blood pressure starts to wear him down. His fatigue comes not from a lack of fitness, but from a disease.

Many times, however, people who improve their fitness level find that their blood pressure drops or some other ailment disappears. So there's a very close interplay between pathological and physiological fatigue.

Mental Fatigue

Mental fatigue is characterized by yawning, sleepiness, and drowsiness. Mental fatigue frequently occurs when doing the same task over and over again. Many writers suffer from mental fatigue after a book is completed. They have taxed their thinking and creative processes to the limit. Many students at the end of the school year are also exhausted mentally.

Generally, though not always, rest and an improvement of physical fitness or nutrition will help solve chronic mental fatigue.

Emotional Fatigue

Emotional fatigue is radically different from physical and mental fatigue. Its causes are insidious, and its cure is complex. Emotional fatigue is usually associated with hurrying, worrying, emotional stress, a fast-paced society, working against the clock, struggling against ill-defined goals, obstacles that seem insurmountable, and change.

Mental and physical fatigue seem to be relieved by rest and a change of some physical condition. Emotional fatigue is another story. The worried executive who tries to sleep his problems away only finds that he sleeps fitfully. And then, when he wakes up, he still feels exhausted. As he dreams he feels he's frustrated, unable to get away from the bear on his back. He dreams one frustrating situation after another. He runs from the enemy but his legs won't move. Conflicts are unresolved. Goals are not achieved. Eighty percent or more of the chronic fatigue problems that people experience are due to emotional fatigue.

Boredom

Many times boredom produces mental fatigue; but it can also precipitate chronic emotional fatigue. In industrialized America many jobs are monotonous. An assembly line job is a perfect example. But even supposedly complex jobs can be boring. A number of physicians have told me that they are bored with the routine of their medical practice: examination after examination after examination.

The problem here is sameness, a lack of stimulation to the brain, nervous and hormonal systems. Extra hormones are not secreted, so a person becomes sleepy and lethargic. That is, unless something out of the ordinary happens. The assembly-line worker becomes alert if the assembly line speeds up. Things would change for me if Michael Jordan walked into my stress-testing lab. And a doctor involved in a life-and-death struggle to save his heart-fibrillating patient will not be bored. When these things happen, we feel full of vim and vigor.

Depression

If you're caught in a state of depression or despondency, you probably also have low levels of energy. Unfortunately, feelings of lost energy tend to feed upon themselves in a vicious, unrelenting cycle. When feeling depressed you experience inertia. You don't want to do anything—physically, mentally, or emotionally. You're not satisfied with the way you're handling life's problems. You become even more depressed. The more depressed you are the more you try to escape reality with sleep. More sleep produces less physical activity and less physical activity produces even lower energy levels. And in turn, these lessened energy levels produce even more depression.

Emotionally drained, you feel depressed. Your self-concept isn't very good either. The depression becomes deeper and the "slow-down" part of your nervous system may become activated. General fatigue sets in. You have very little energy, if any. Soon you start to experience anger. Because your self-concept isn't what it should be, you repress it.

Anger

Anger is another problem. As it stimulates your nervous system, blood pressure rises, heart rate increases, and hormones are secreted.

Venting your spleen in anger offers good news and bad news. The good news is that you probably dissipate your emotions and relax your muscle tension. The bad news is that the recipient of your outburst may lash back at you, only serving to heighten your anger and create a greater sympathetic response on your part. While arguing you may be full of energy, but afterwards you feel whipped because of the tremendous emotional-physical strain placed on your body. A second part of the bad news may be that the recipient of your outburst is hurt, producing feelings of guilt on your part that only add to your stress.

Repression of your anger doesn't work here either. Your muscles are tense, your blood pressure is high, sugar is secreted, and extra hormones are circulating in your bloodstream. You're fighting like mad to keep the emotions inside. Suddenly you feel tired. Emotionally drained. You retire to bed or to sleep. You toss and turn. Sleep finally comes. But it's not truly restful. You awaken exhausted. Your nervous system again wants to act, but you put a damper on it. You're still angry but you don't do anything about it. Now you become depressed.

The body interrupts all of this and uses its protective mechanism of depression to help you handle your angry feelings. You have felt so much stimulation, so much anger, and so much hostility, that the only way you can protect your body is by shutting down. The result is an extremely low level of energy. But you don't read it as that. You read it as an inability to control your life and feelings.

Slowly your self-concept slips, and more depression occurs. The deeper the depression, the more inertia. Soon a vicious cycle of anger, depression, inertia, poor-self-concept, back to anger is set up. And you don't give a damn about anything.

Of course, other emotions such a guilt and jealousy are also kept inside and probably produce a similar response to anger. In fact, the guilt and jealousy probably cause you to be angrier still, and the same cycle starts again.

Anxiety

Anxiety is closely allied with depression. Oftentimes, a person is anxious first and as the anxiety builds and heightens it progresses into depression. Depression, quite frankly, is the circuit breaker for anxiety. Anxiety-producing situations cause people to get more and more whipped up. They keep taking on more and more input of fear, anticipation of something stressful, and worry. They become more and more apprehensive. Soon the anxiety interferes with their ability to concentrate. That is followed by psychosomatic symptoms which produce more anxiety. Hormone levels skyrocket. The body rebels and starts to shut down. Depression follows. They then become anxious about depression.

The anxiety, depression, and back to anxiety circle occurs simply because the internal balance of the hormonal and nervous systems has been disrupted. Soon their body is caught in an overload. To protect the body, the various systems shut down and the person becomes depressed. The result is less and less energy.

Emotional fatigue causes a sensory overload, taking your mind, body, and emotions beyond your ability to cope. Research done by the National Institute of Mental Health illustrates this point. Experiments with an electroencephalogram indicate that the brain controls a "sensoristat" that helps us control the effects of sensory stimulation. When you are overstimulated emotionally, this mechanism dials down to prevent an overload. If you are exposed to high levels of pressure, responsibility, and change, the sensoristat dims your perception to protect you. And that response results in feelings of lethargy and fatigue. Often, such an overload brings about total collapse. More often, however, it creates that frustrating feeling of not having enough steam to get through the day.

An Old Body in a Brave New World

In many ways, we are a lot like prehistoric human. When he was attacked by an animal or another human his nerves and glands would make necessary adjustments to improve his chances for survival. The grey matter of his brain told him that danger was imminent and signaled the hypothalamus—that small, specialized tissue that is the key to many bodily adjustments. The hypothalamus, in turn, relayed the same message to the nervous and endocrine systems. The key centers activated were the sympathetic nervous system (the stimulating part of the autonomic nervous system), and the pituitary gland.

Still Fighting Saber-toothed Tigers

Today, our bodies have inherited the same mechanisms. When we are faced with stress our hypothalamus is stimulated and our sympathetic nervous system and hormones swing into action. But instead of saber-toothed tigers and invading barbarians, we are confronted by crowds, job frustrations, domestic responsibilities, social demands, and change. Although these challenges are mental in nature, our brain perceives them as dangerous. The message it sends to the body is the same one a caveman would have received: fight or flight.

Unfortunately, our response today is short-circuited. First, we don't know who or where the enemy is. Second, we have many potential stresses hitting us at one time. Third, we don't know how to respond to our enemies, or we have been chastised since childhood to keep feelings and emotions inside. So we internalize our frustrations, anxieties, and hostility. It is not socially acceptable to run away from the office or to punch the ulcer-producing boss in the nose when we fail to meet his standards. Instead, we passively sit and take it, though sitting on our feelings and not doing something physical is counter to our heritage. Immobilization in attitude and action causes significant problems because first, we are not fit enough to handle the pressure; and second, the sitting produces a nervous and endocrine response that is not dissipated as it should be.

In earlier times, man lived by his strength and endurance. Every task required the vigorous use of his body. Success in life meant being able to run fast and long and to strike hard if attacked. Fitness was necessary for survival. As man progressed, he started to use tools and animals, and his work became a little easier. Still, man's brawn had to be used if he was to survive.

Eventually a dramatic change occurred. The Industrial Revolution brought a way of life alien to man. The automobile became king. People moved to suburbia, shopping centers sprang up, and interstate highways connected cities.

Stress Has Changed, We Haven't

Today, actual physical labor is almost nonexistent. Modern technology has created a lifestyle in which the great majority of people in industrialized societies do little physical work—at home or on the job. So our fitness slips; our fitness to fight or our fitness to handle stress.

Interestingly, this problem is not seen in primitive societies, where threats to life and security more often come in physical forms that demand direct, physical responses. Threatened by hunger, thirst, natural phenomena, or enemies, the people in nontechnological societies act naturally to avert the threat, and the action discharges the stored energy before it has a chance to accumulate and cause severe emotional fatigue. The primitive may be tired physically, but he does not have physical fatigue due to emotional wipeout.

One frightening experience (a near accident), an argument with the boss, or a disappointing performance will not insult your body. You are tougher than that! But the constant pressure of a bad marriage, a poor relationship with your children, a hated job, and a list of other conflicts can and will cause the body (particularly the sympathetic nervous and endocrine systems) to be overworked, and cause overstimulation. This overstimulation manifests itself with physical, mental, and especially emotional fatigue.

Early man had an option that most of us don't use to advantage. He was a physical person. That helped him cope. As much as we hate to admit it, we are no longer physical people, regardless of today's fitness boom. Though many Americans picture themselves as active, most are not. Scientists have been able to demonstrate that. They've been able to show that the fitness levels of North Americans have declined. They also know that once a basic level of fitness is lost, there is little you can do to fight stress and to have the energy to survive unless you rebuild your fitness level.

Research on Fitness

North Americans are fatigued because of a lack of fitness. Dr. Donald Bailey (University of Saskatchewan), along with Dr. Roy Shephard (University of Toronto), tested 672 women and 558 men to find their fitness levels. The results? These Canadian men and women tested poorly. And the women were somewhat worse than the men. The least fit group of all was young women in their 20's.

There's no reason to expect U.S. citizens would fare any better. In fact, small studies done at various locations in the United States suggest we may be less fit.

A primary reason for the decline in fitness levels is that we are not active physically. Look at these facts: Back in the 1930's, the average American male expended 3,000 calories a day. The average female expended 2,400. Today, the average American male burns off 2,200 calories a day and the average female 1,500. That means 800 to 900 calories of activity per day have been programmed out of our lives: that is equivalent to the energy expended during an eight- or nine-mile jog. The bottom line is, of course, that we do not work as hard physically as our predecessors. The result is overwhelming fatigue. We are too tired to get through the day because we don't have the energy reserve that comes from fitness.

The American Way to Decreased Energy

It is a simple fact that the American way of life begets fatigue and a feeling of no energy, and one of the biggest problems is a lack of physical fitness. Despite all the hoopla and attention focused on fitness in this country, the number of Americans who exercise regularly is low.

Most experts agree that regular exercise is participation in any activity at least three times a week. Work by the President's Council on Physical Fitness and Sports has shown that a large percentage of our adult population does not sufficiently exercise. Most people who do exercise participate only two days a week or less.

The President's Council has indicated that only 30 million Americans exercise regularly, about 20 percent of our population. Furthermore, they have stated that 45 percent of the population gets no exercise at all! Other experts see the situation as being even more dismal.

Dr. Kenneth Cooper, of aerobics fame, believes the President's Council's estimate that 30 million Americans exercise regularly is an enormous exaggeration. "It's probably more like 10 to 15 million—probably less—and even those people aren't exercising regularly."

The most skeptical of all, however, is Dr. Joseph Ahrens, a cardiologist specializing in preventive medicine. He states that "past the age of 35 less than 2 percent of American males and less than 1 percent of American females are physically fit." In other words, only 1 to 2 percent of those people past the age of 35 are getting adequate exercise.

The phenomenon of lack of physical activity is shown in the rapid increase of obesity. Of at least 10 million teenagers, 2 out of 10 are overweight. Among adults, 3 out of 10 men and 4 out of 10 women over 40 are more than 20 percent above their ideal weight. Seat manufacturers tell us that they now design broader-bottomed chairs for our broader-bottomed citizens. Clothing manufacturers report that both sexes and all ages have shown an increase in arm, chest, and body measurements.

Not only are we fat, we seem to be getting fatter. A weight gain of a pound each year after age 25 is considered "normal" by most physicians. That means a 150-pound, 25-year-old person can expect to weigh 190 pounds by the time he retires. It's little wonder the good things he never had time for—playing with the kids, outdoor sports, dancing, sex—are now out of his feeble, flabby reach.

Eating More, Getting Less

Additionally, some experts feel that the food we eat, the very stuff that's supposed to provide us with energy, is a major energy-robber and a significant contributor to the fatigue problem. Today, the primary criteria for judging a meal seems to be speed: If it can be done in 15 minutes or less, that's good. If it takes time, that's bad. Unfortunately, speed comes in boxes, cans, and metal trays—more salt, sugar, and fat, and not much in the way of vitamins, minerals, and complex carbohydrates.

A simple illustration is the potato. Give most people a choice and they'll ask for french fries over baked. The reason? "I can eat it with my fingers." "I don't have time to prepare a baked potato." "I can take 'em right out of a bag and pop them in the oven." "French fries taste better." Yet, by the time a serving of french fries has been thawed from a long term in the freezer, boiled in a vat of grease, and then sprinkled with more salt than a human needs in a week, the potato has gained over 100 calories and lost a good bit of its nutrition.

Contributing to this nutrition problem is the absence of fresh foods from our diets. Since our lifestyle does not allow for daily shopping at a fresh-food market, we rely greatly on canned or frozen foods. Consequently, we end up eating some fiber (which is good) but very little nutrition. For example, peas lose 38 percent of their vitamins in the canning process and 27 percent in the freezing process. By the time you eat a frozen dinner it has lost 40 percent of the vitamin A, 100 percent of the vitamin C, 80 percent of the B complex vitamins, and 55 percent of the vitamin E. It's like pouring low-octane gasoline into the fuel tank of a high-performance automobile. The engine just doesn't have the pep because the fuel is deficient.

Probably the biggest culprit in the nutrition scam is sugar. Sugar is everywhere. If you don't believe me, grab any food item packaged in a box. Sugar is almost always listed in the ingredients, which are listed by weight. Such sneak attacks of sugar on the American diet have resulted in an annual consumption of 120 pounds of sugar per person.

What's so bad about sugar? I'll discuss that more in Chapter 12, but briefly, sugar has been implicated in disease conditions that cause some people to have a drastic loss of energy. Many people who experience the feeling of being run down, run out, or run over have a sugar metabolism problem, a condition which falls into a category that could be described as "the slows."

When it comes to surviving in this brave new world of ours we are clobbered. We are caught in the midst of a rapidly changing world that stresses us with fast-paced living, changing values, and ill-defined roles. And most of us are not fit enough to survive in this world. We are sedentary and eat foods which deplete our energy. Years ago, only the fittest survived the onslaughts of nature. Today, only the fittest can make it through this maze of future shock. If you want to enjoy this life to the fullest, if you want to maximize your personal energy, if you want the true pleasure of living at the capacity that is optimal for you, you must take charge and become fit.

We'll Do Anything for a Rush

Some of the very things people use to obtain energy become negative, energy-reducing addictions. We have become a society that looks to everyone and everything else for the solution to our energy problems. We smoke, even though we know it's not good for us. We consume too much alcohol, even though it strains relationships, decreases productivity, and reduces personal effectiveness. We use drugs—over-the-counter, prescription, and illegal substances—even though the potential for irreparable harm is frightening. Even our sources of entertainment have become an inescapable trap.

What is it that compels us to become hooked on these self-destructive preoccupations? It would probably take a roomful of psychiatrists to come up with a thorough answer, but it is my belief that part of the problem lies in our endless search for stimulation. We want a rush, a lift, to help us through the day. We'll do just about anything to get a surge of adrenaline. And often, the things we do are at best energy-robbing, and even life-threatening.

Smoking

If smoking were similar to taking vitamins or grabbing a handful of peanuts occasionally, no one would be worried. But we are worried. By the 1940's doctors began to notice an alarming increase in deaths due to lung cancer. Without a great deal of research they were able to correlate this increase with cigarette smoking. Later, they found an association between smoking and many other diseases, such as heart disease and bladder cancer. Currently, the dangers of smoking are printed on every pack and the government has conducted a media blitz that condemns the use of cigarettes. We have been given every reason to avoid cigarettes, yet people continue to smoke. Why?

It starts with peer pressure. While kids may no longer go behind the barn to sneak a few puffs, most people get started as youngsters, who succumb to the need to be accepted by their friends who think that smoking is the adult thing to do. Soon, however, they find that they need to smoke. Ask a person why she lights up first thing in the morning and she'll say, "It wakes me up." Ask him why he smokes after supper and he'll say, "It relaxes me." As incongruous as it may seem, smoking seems to do both.

First, the nicotine in smoke reacts with the acetylcholine receptors of the brain. Acetylcholine is a nerve transmitter in the brain. This interaction causes the autonomic nervous system to respond. The nicotine causes extra adrenaline to be secreted. As a result, there's an increase in blood pressure, heart rate, cardiac output, and blood sugar level. In other words, a smoker gets a rush, a surge of energy, albeit nervous energy.

Shortly after that initial lift, however, the body tends to slow down. And that explains how cigarettes can have a calming effect. In essence, the smoker is strangling himself. Any time a person inhales smoke he's ingesting carbon monoxide, which prevents smokers from getting the usual amount of life-giving oxygen. The general slowing-down effect of smoking is really a subtle energy drain, hence a sense of relaxation. Instead of actually calming down and relaxing, a smoker is merely pulling the plug on his energy supply. Repeated smoking adds to this depletion of energy. Just as the body starts to slow down, the smoker feels he needs a lift. One puff and he stimulates his body again. But soon the body must rest and fatigue sets in. As a result, when a smoker lights up to fight fatigue he's really beating a dead horse. And, if you're the smoker, the dead horse is you.

Alcohol

But smoking isn't enough. In our quest for more and more stimulation we turn to alcohol. Initially, there is nothing more stimulating than a couple of drinks. We have convinced ourselves that everything from hobbies to parties are more enjoyable with a can or glass in one of our hands.

The problem with this line of thinking is that alcohol's lift is promptly followed by a depressing slow-down of the person's entire system. In fact, alcohol is classified by the medical profession not as a stimulant, but as a depressant. The initial surge of energy you get from a drink or two is rather short-lived. In a short period of time you're going to feel tired and irritable. If you were in the proper setting, you would probably fall asleep for an energy-building catnap. Unfortunately, most people drink in settings that do not allow a nap—during lunch hour, at a bar, or at a party in another part of town. The tired feeling many people experience after a drink or two may be due to a sludging of the blood cells. Hence, less energy-giving oxygen is carried to the body's cells—especially the brain cells. The end product is fatigue.

The Pill Generation

Never before have Americans of all ages consumed so many sleeping pills, pep pills, diet pills, sedatives, and tranquilizers. They have been convinced that anything can be cured by the right pharmaceutical concoction.

There are some people who take a pill every morning to clear the cobwebs, and take another every evening to help them sleep. Still others take pills to lose weight or pills to reduce anxiety. Drugs have become a way of life. We turn to them for assistance instead of learning to handle our problems in a mature, self-reliant manner.

Amphetamines are used by millions of Americans for stimulation. Speed hypes you up with nervous energy for a very concrete reason. It increases the activity of hormones that heighten brain activity and makes a person so jittery that the user cannot sit still. If the amphetamine hype is unsatisfactory, cocaine is frequently the drug of choice. These drugs will definitely give you a lift. But the after-effects of their use are severe fatigue and lethargy. Possible side effects are forms of psychosis.

Why do we use them? To get stimulation, to get a lift, a rise, to overcome fatigue, the blahs, and burn-out. We want energy. We have more confidence in a chemical than in our own ability to control our energy. In essence, we have admitted we can't do anything about our problems.

In our search for stimulation, we have allowed tobacco, alcohol, and other mood-altering drugs to become our masters. The tragedy is the admission that we are nothing without the help of a chemical friend. Life is exciting only when we have something artificial to give us a boost. That mind set carries into our entire outlook on life and creates a society interested in more and more of whatever turns us on. Even the things we do for enjoyment have become infected with this self-deprecating philosophy.

The All-American Way

Vicariously, we try to experience the ultimate high of winning the World Series with the bases-loaded, bottom-of-the-ninth home run, or playing at a sold-out Madison Square Garden rock concert. And it all starts with the natural desire to find more energy. Let me illustrate.

In the 1950's, television began to shape the American way of life. Evening meals were scheduled around "Uncle Miltie" and "Our Miss Brooks." By the 1960's, 90 percent of American homes had a TV to show them, among other things, morning films of the previous night's Vietnam battles, followed by Captain Kangaroo. A full 98 percent of our households boasted of at least one television by the 1970's and it was estimated that average school children watched 3 1/2 hours each day and saw over 250,000 commercials by the time they graduated from high school. If you go back and examine the content of programming over those 40 years, you will notice that each season tries to outdo the last in terms of action.

I do not intend to moralize, but rather to illustrate the extent to which television has programmed our thinking. In our quest for stimulation, we have developed an insatiable desire for more. There may be nothing inherently wrong with a soap opera or situation comedy. There is something drastically wrong, however, when that show becomes a fix, mainlining a quick kick to us to get us through the day. Whenever we have to go outside of ourselves for stimulation, we lay ourselves wide open to negative addiction, which could lead to decreased energy. A lifestyle dominated by television viewing can hardly be described as energetic.

A Nation of Spectators

Of course, television isn't the only culprit. The need to be stimulated is one reason why spectator-sport attendance remains high even during depressed economic times. Hold on a minute, you say! A day at the old ball park can be a great energizing experience. Here in the Midwest, a favorite fall pastime is a tailgate picnic in the parking lot of a football stadium followed by an exciting collegiate football game. I'm all for it.

Yet there is a side to spectator sports that is becoming increasingly ugly: the thirst for violence. Any auto racing promoter will tell you the best way to assure a packed grandstand is to have an occasional spectacular crash. People are repelled by the sight of blood at a boxing match, but tickets are selling better than ever. Each baseball season seems to provide more bench-clearing brawls than ever before. And football? Deacon Jones, former rampaging defensive end for the Los Angeles Rams, said, "Football is meant to be a violent sport, that's what makes it so popular. People want blood. They want toughness. They want violence..." The obvious answer to the question, "What's next?" was answered frighteningly a number of years ago in yet another form of entertainment. The movie Rollerball graphically portrayed a society of thrill-seekers queuing up at box offices to see a new breed of athletes physically annihilate one another.

Other forms of entertainment have fallen into this pattern of one-upmanship. Depending on which way you look at it, music has come a long way since the days of baroque chamber recitals and concert hall decorum. Perhaps Elvis set the pace with his undulating lower torso, but he was soon outdone by rock acts that feature performers who demonstrate behavior with emphasis upon sadism, masochism, and general vulgarity. In film, slow-motion, stop-action conventional killing has become old hat. Now, slow-motion, stop action unconventional killing is in vogue.

Regardless of the moral label that you place on modern culture, when you become hopelessly addicted to the role of a spectator, two things happen. First, you have denied yourself the opportunity to be your own stimulating, energizing agent. You have, in effect, declared, "I can no longer find energy in things that I do, only in things that I sit back and watch." You become increasingly vulnerable to the syndrome that causes you to keep chasing thrills until there's nothing left to outdo the last one. The result is a pervasive form of boredom that typifies nonenergetic people. Nothing turns them on any more, hence a loss of drive and the resolve to do anything but exist with the faint hope that something thrilling will happen someday.

The Materialism Trap

When television fails to provide the stimulus you need, turn it off and turn on your snowmobile, or powerboat, or 4-wheel-drive stump-jumper. It's as much as to say, "Give me enough things and I'll be happy."

The materialism trap is based on the premise that nothing satisfies. Yet is begins with that dangerous assumption, "If I only had one of those small, nylon backpacking tents and some hiking boots, I'd really be happy." After a few camping trips with this equipment, you opt for the mountaineering model complete with floor and zippered bug screen. The next year, it's a camper, and of course, to pull it you need a bigger car. A few years after that and you may buy a self-contained, air-conditioned, fully carpeted, motor home complete with wet bar and dishwasher. And secretly you're dreaming of owning a private mountain resort.

Indeed, the entire American way of life is programmed toward the accumulation of things, not for the sake of utility, but for the pleasure we get from owning. Few people buy a car with the intention of driving it until it quits running. We buy every two or three years because new cars look better, sound better, and smell better. Similarly, we seldom wear clothes until they wear out. We buy clothes to keep up with the styles. Yet the real irony is the end result. Those who live in a simpler, less materialistic culture often are happier, better adjusted, and more energetic people. Those who spend the least amount of time chasing after happiness seem to find it and enjoy it more.

Ours is a culture that leaps at any opportunity to be stimulated. We grope from one fix to the next, hoping to find that elusive, ultimate trip. Our habits of smoking and drinking don't provide it. Our forms of entertainment promise it but never deliver. The things we play with offer little relief from the lethargic boredom that grips us. Yet we keep trying, keep reaching, distraught, dissatisfied, unhappy, and out of gas.

The answer?

Our best source of energy is ourselves. We have the physical and emotional capabilities to live lives with a maximum of energy, if we are willing to capitalize on our own abilities and make use of current information on building energy.

▶▶▶ *Section II:* ▶▶▶

Your Energy Quotient

Pure Energy ▶▶**5**▶▶

E veryone claims you must get your energy from some outside source. A panty hose ad used to sing "sheer energy." A breakfast cereal touted "go power." A beverage company promised their soda would leave you "feelin' good." But you have read the first four chapters of this book and no longer believe their claims. Now you're hoping I'll give you the facts, the real stuff of energy, the answers.

And I will, but first I need to explain—your American way of living isn't the only factor to consider in assessing your energy level. The other factor is the body you were born with and the internal energy that came with it. To understand energy you must see the phenomenon of your physiology and body chemistry. You must understand what you have to work with to maximize your personal energy.

The Brain

Some experts believe that you get your energy potential from your brain's chemicals and structure, which is largely dictated by your genes. Your brain is truly amazing. It weighs slightly more than three pounds and has about 100 billion nerve cells. These extremely tiny nerve cells look like a lop-sided spider. Extending from the cell body are spiderlike arms called "dendrites." The single long arm is an "axon." The axon's length can be anywhere from a fraction of a millimeter to well over one yard long. These nerve cells with long and short arms are so densely packed and intertwined in your brain that it looks like an electrician's nightmare.

The axons, however, interface with the dendrites of other nerve cells. They are not fastened together, but are separated by a microscopic gap called a synapse. These many nerve cells with dendrites and axons serve as a communications network for the brain and your nervous system. They help transmit impulses throughout the brain quickly and efficiently via a relay mechanism.

A Special Relay Team

When a relay team races, each runner passes a baton to the next runner in what trackmen call a passing zone. Your neurons, dendrites, synapses, and axons act like a relay team, passing an impulse rather than a baton.

During the passage of the nerve impulse, rapid electrochemical changes take place along the nerve. The impulse travels from the dendrites toward the axon. When the impulse gets to the end of the axon it must pass over the gap or synapse to the next cell's dendrites. The synapse is much like the passing zone in the relay race. To make the jump between the axon of one nerve and the dendrite of another, a chemical is released that permits the impulse to travel across the synapse. As soon as the impulse is across the synapse, another chemical is released and destroys the activity of the first chemical. This release and destruction of chemicals allows for only one message to be transmitted at a time, but the relay pass is successful and the race continues on to the spinal cord, brain, or muscles. All this happens extremely fast.

Nerve Transmitters

The chemicals that transmit the impulse from nerve cell to nerve cell are called nerve transmitters. Many nerve transmitters have been discovered and probably many more will be found in the future.

As you would suspect, these various nerve transmitters are not secreted randomly. Instead, selected nerve cells secrete only one kind of transmitter, such as dopamine, acetylcholine, epinephrine, norepinephrine, or serotonin. By secreting only one kind of chemical the electrical impulse finds its way throughout the maze of cells in the brain. These nerve transmitters make road maps or blueprints for the electrical impulse and the resulting action. Actions include: thinking, talking, walking, singing, loving, writing, moving, hating, and enjoying—in other words, enjoying and celebrating life.

Over the years, scientists have isolated the role of the known chemicals.

They know norepinephrine plays a role in dreaming and in your emotions. Dopamine helps you to make coordinated movements.

These nerve transmitters also play a role in your energy levels. Experts tell us that mood swings occur because of too much or not enough chemicals being secreted. For example, if your brain produces too much norepinephrine you may be moved to uncontrollable rage. Likewise, too little production of this chemical may cause the blues or depression.

Of course, mood swings are much more complex than the secretion of one or two chemicals. It is conceivable that selected nerve cells may be oversensitive to certain chemicals. Or the brain may produce the right amount of norepinephrine but the chemical is not removed quickly enough from the synapse. It is also possible that mood shifts may be dependent upon the intensity of the "electrical" surge across the synapse or along the axon.

Regardless of the reason, it can be safely stated that, to a point, your inborn energy levels are dictated by chemicals, electrical impulses, and various nerve cells. Consequently, you may have very high or low energy levels simply because you may or may not secrete a certain amount of nerve transmitters.

The Nervous System

The nervous system itself also plays an important role in your energy levels. Your autonomic nervous system is composed of two systems. The parasympathetic nervous system keeps you calm, cool, and collected. It keeps your blood pressure and heart rate low, reduces the secretion of various hormones, and keeps you on an even keel. In other words, it dampens your emotions and reactions.

The sympathetic nervous system, on the other hand, heightens your response to life's events. It increases your heart rate and blood pressure. It releases blood sugar into your bloodstream. It secretes extra amounts of hormones so you can fight for longer periods of time and it speeds up your metabolic rate.

In general, your sympathetic nervous system keeps you wide awake, vital, and full of energy. The activation of the sympathetic nervous system can be good for heightened energy.

Without your sympathetic nervous system you would not be able to make love. The winning of a football game could not be savored. There would be little desire or motivation to excel. But if the sympathetic system is activated too often and too long, it can be bad for your energy levels as I will explain later. A fine balance must be kept between the stimulation of the sympathetic and the parasympathetic nervous system for maximum personal energy.

Your brain and nervous system, however, aren't the only sources of energy lifts or letdowns. The endocrine or hormonal system plays a crucial role as well.

The Pituitary Gland

The pituitary gland, only about 1/2 inch in diameter and located at the base of your brain, has a profound effect on your energy. It activates other glands to action. It also secretes many hormones that influence growth and skin color, but I'll only concentrate on those pituitary hormones that raise or lower your level of energy.

The pituitary gland secretes ACTH or adrenocorticotropic hormone. ACTH stimulates the adrenal cortex, which activates cortisol, a hormone that has a direct effect on your energy. When you are anticipating a stressful or exciting event, your adrenals will secrete more cortisol. Cortisol levels increase when you're waiting for a test to begin, anticipating your first airplane ride, or getting ready to descend a roller coaster chute. When the event takes place, your cortisol level drops and other hormones take over. Cortisol levels change throughout the day. Concentrate hard to meet a deadline, or experience an upsetting event such as an argument, or go through an unsure situation, and your cortisol levels will rise. Conversely, when everything seems in synchronization, your cortisol level will drop.

The secretion of cortisol prepares you for the impending event by sharpening your senses. By sharpening your senses, you are able to fully appreciate the activity. You have greater feelings of energy. Without cortisol our world and life would be dull, dull, dull.

The pituitary gland also secretes thyrotropic—the thyroid-stimulating hormone (TSH). TSH regulates the size and structure of the thyroid and stimulates the production of thyroxine.

Thyroxine

Tyroxine has a profound effect upon your energy levels. Thyroxine affects what doctors call your metabolism, the speed with which your body's cells burn the food that you have digested and the oxygen that your body takes in. Each cell is dependent upon oxygen and selected food nutrients to perform its duty, whether that duty is contraction by muscle cells, thinking and reasoning by brain cells, or the transmission of impulses by nerve cells.

If a lot of it is secreted, thyroxine allows the cells of your body to utilize oxygen and nutrients very rapidly. Hence, your metabolism is high. People who have excessive thyroxine tend to feel jittery, and have a rapid heart rate and increased blood pressure. If the body releases excessively low amounts of thyroxine, the opposite occurs: listlessness lethargy.

Normally, thyroxine production is fairly constant and only under stress, pressure, or something similar does your pituitary gland stimulate your thyroid gland to produce more thyroxine. Hence, one of the reasons you feel hyper or jittery during a speech, athletic event, or during an argument is because of your thyroxine level. Much like cortisol, without thyroxine your life would be boring. These hormones allow you to enjoy life to its fullest.

Some people, however, have a permanently malfunctioning thyroid gland. Consequently, they are listless or jittery all the time, depending upon whether their body produces too little or too much of the hormone. An underactive thyroid gland that does not secrete enough thyroxine makes the metabolism very slow. Since food is not used at a proper rate, the person becomes fat. An underactive thyroid also produces a feeling of listlessness. The person is not lazy, he just doesn't have the energy to move.

An underactive thyroid of this type occurs in only about 2 percent of obese people. Consequently, if you have a weight-gain problem, you should not surmise that it's due to a sluggish thyroid. It's probably due to a sedentary lifestyle and improper eating habits.

An overactive thyroid can also cause problems. Here the body burns food too rapidly, causing loss of weight and excessive appetite. Other signs of the disease are nervousness, insomnia, and dizziness. In some instances the eyes bulge and give a person a staring look. Sweating when you should be cold is another symptom. Also, sometimes the thyroid gland becomes enlarged.

There are several factors affecting thyroid production. Some people may be born with a defective gland, or a tumor may appear. It's possible that there may not be enough iodine in the diet. But other reasons are also recognized. Worry, fear, anxiety, and other emotional stresses and strains may be factors. These stress factors can stimulate the production of the thyroid hormone. As a result, the thyroid can be overworked. The extra stimulation may cause the thyroid to become overactive, and then after a while, it gives up.

You may know people on some kind of thyroid medication. Sometime, ask them how they feel. Many will tell you that immediately after taking thyroxine they feel a rush of energy, followed by a hyped-up feeling. They're jittery. Their pulse rates may be 130 or more beats per minute. As their day wears on, however, the thyroxine level is somewhat modulated and they gradually settle down. Near the end of the day, or 24 hours later, the effectiveness of the medication wanes and they start to feel lethargic. That is why most people on thyroxine pills take their medication early in the day. They get the sudden lift early in the morning, much like people get with coffee. Then, throughout the day they experience more normal levels. They sleep when the thyroxine levels are lowest, at night.

Other Pituitary Hormones

The pituitary secretes two other hormones as well: ADH (an anti-diuretic) and vasopressin. Both of these hormones can raise blood pressure. Increased blood pressure for an emergency may be good, but if increased for an extended period of time, it may adversely affect energy levels in a rather strange way. Experts theorize that the fatigue which usually accompanies high blood pressure patients may be caused by the body's attempt to lower the pressure since blood pressures tend to drop with rest.

The Adrenal Gland

The adrenal gland secretes a hormone called epinephrine, sometimes called adrenaline. Adrenaline increases blood sugar and speeds up the heart. It can increase the metabolic rate 150 percent or more. People who are given a shot of synthetic adrenaline feel a tremendous rush of energy. They feel capable of doing things they normally couldn't do and become extremely hyper and jittery.

Your own adrenaline can cause you to respond in the same way. When the adrenal glands are stimulated by fear, anger, anxiety, or excitement, an "adrenaline high" is produced. The amount of adrenaline secreted by your adrenal glands is dictated by heredity and the severity of the real or imagined threat.

When adrenaline is released, you feel wide awake, alert, and raring to go. Many athletes, by concentrating on the event and their competition, "psych themselves up" for the event. In other words, they're able to deliberately increase their adrenaline levels.

Your Biological Clock

Each individual seems to have a timing device within that increases or decreases their supply of energy. That may sound rather complicated, but people's inner clocks differ just as larks, which are active in the day, differ from owls, which are active at night. Allow me to illustrate.

My wife, Beth, is a late evening person, an owl. I'm an early morning person, a lark. The most creative part of the day for me is before noon. I like to be up by five or six o'clock in the morning because I know my energy levels will be really cranked up. I leave my perfunctory tasks for the afternoon because my motivation and drive is way down. Beth, on the other hand, is just starting to rev her engines by the time I'm winding down. She is extremely energetic in the evening and seems to enjoy more energy as midnight approaches. The next morning, however, she has to start slowly because her level of energy is down.

Everyone has such a clock within them, and no one's sure why. The limited research in the area suggests that part of it is inborn and part of it is learned. As far as I'm concerned, that's not the important part. It's far more important that you know when your body produces its greatest amount of energy and try to arrange your activities around the highs and lows. If you are an owl, save your creative work for the evening. If you are a lark, don't try to accomplish major tasks in the late afternoon. By getting your work and activity load in "sync" with your biological clock, you will more fully utilize your energy potential.

The interplay of your nervous system, brain, and hormonal systems illustrates quite clearly how your body can be energized internally. It demonstrates how you can activate resources within your body to increase or decrease your energy levels.

You might be thinking, "This is all very interesting, but what can I do about it?" The answer is, not much. You could go to your doctor and have tests taken to determine how much of which hormones you secrete when. But there is little sense in that. I don't recommend taking any drugs to supplement your hormone production unless you have exhausted the suggestions given in the rest of this book. Relying on medication slips you back into dependency on some exterior source. It also could quickly become a serious negative addiction that would throw your system completely out of whack. It is conceivable that your hormones are the source of your energy problem, but I doubt it. Instead, consider the other possible options.

Your Life Space ▶▶**6**▶▶

Two Stories

The year was 1928. Hulda Crooks was tired, and I mean tired. She had just finished several grueling years in which she had moved from her rural farm in Canada, belatedly finished her high school education, attended Loma Linda University in California, and received her degree in dietetics. In addition to this intense activity, she had worked her way through both high school and college.

She also had married Dr. Samuel A. Crooks, instructor of anatomy at Loma Linda University. She was in love. But she was also pooped. "He literally took me for better or worse," she confided. Working for her college degree had worn her out. She remembers, "I wasn't worth much. I was nervous, anemic, and perpetually tired. As I worked for my support and education, year after year of indoor life took its toll. So, although I gained an education I lost my health and energy. I was so tired, I was afraid I would die." She was only in her late 20's.

Hulda's new husband started her on a plan to help her regain energy and vitality. She was to spend as much time outdoors as possible, gardening and raising lovebirds, calves, and goats. She was also to improve her mind, develop a positive attitude about life, and follow a healthful, vegetarian eating plan. At first she could barely walk around the block. But as time progressed she was able to walk for miles, and work for hours in the yard.

As Hulda's strength and vitality started to return she began to do more demanding things. Backpacking and mountain climbing became a way of life. Expeditions would last from one to six weeks. Vacations were spent at altitudes of 11,000 feet. She began to run at the age of 70. In time, she was running distances of up to a half marathon (13.1 miles).

By the time I met and interviewed Hulda she was 84 years old and far from ready for the rocking chair. She was sweet, alert, vibrant, and energetic, a real "possibility" thinker. As we chatted, she told me that she was still an avid backpacker. She had climbed Mt. Whitney 18 times in 18 years. In 1972 she crossed the Sierra Nevada range from Sequoia to Whitney Portal—an 80-mile trip.

I left her small apartment feeling good about life, getting older, and people. I was energized.

Turning Back the Clock

Steve McKanic had also virtually run out of steam. After 22 years of building a fuel oil delivery business, his lifestyle had caught up with him. Skipping breakfast, gulping coffee, smoking 3 1/2 packs of cigarettes a day, and working 18-hour days had just about done him in. Each day he found it more and more difficult to drag himself out of bed and off to work. Finally, the "big one" hit and laid him flat in a hospital. The prognosis was bleak. His heart was too diseased for bypass surgery. Two cardiologists at separate medical schools told him, "No hope. Go home, get your things in order. At most you have six months to live. In fact, if you want to live that long, take this medication and stay in bed."

Steve's back was to the wall and he knew it. At first, he moped around the house cursing his fate. He spent a lot of time "if only-ing." You know, "If only I had taken it easier. If only I had gone on a diet." When he tired of that, he made a decision. If he was going to die it would be in the saddle, not in a rocking chair.

He began reading intensely about heart disease, to learn what he could do. His conclusion was to fight back by doing the following:
- Develop a positive attitude about life
- Lose 80 pounds
- Stop smoking 3 1/2 packs of cigarettes a day
- Begin exercising
- Improve eating habits: Decrease fat, sugar, and salt; and supplement the diet with vitamins and minerals

Gradually, Steve became a new person. One night he even went for a walk. He did it late at night so no one could see him. His wife was upset. At the end of the walk he was mildly surprised that nothing happened. So he went for another walk the next day, fully expecting to drop dead. He didn't, so he continued the next, and the next, and the next. The more he walked the better he felt. Over the months, he moved up to walking and jogging 10 to 11 miles a day. This gave him more energy than he'd ever thought possible. His weight started to drop. His nutrition improved dramatically.

Steve didn't stop with these efforts. He spent eight hours a day for a year studying how to improve his health. At a local college he took courses in nutrition, fitness, psychology, and stress management. He also started to share his newfound information with friends and strangers. When someone had a heart attack he visited them in the hospital and told them there was hope, or could be, if they began assuming responsibility for their own health. He encouraged them to get the most out of what they had left *and* never give up.

Steve lived for more than seven years after his April 1973 heart attack. He told me just before his death in July 1980 that the last seven years of his life were his best. He gave and received more energy, fun, and love during those years than all of his previous 47 years combined. Steve was special, and he illustrates an important point: even if you already have one foot in the grave, it's not too late to achieve your maximum remaining energy potential.

Creating Your Own Energy Story

These stories are important. You simply must not count yourself too old or too far gone to do something about your lack of healthful energy. So let's begin with today—now.

The first thing you must do is accept responsibility for your own behavior, feelings, actions, and attitudes. You can change your actions—if you decide to do so.

The hardest thing you will do is overcome immobilization. Here are some examples.

- You don't exercise because you're afraid you won't have the time.
- You want to exercise but are afraid people will laugh at you.
- You want to eat salad at noon but are afraid your associates will make fun of your "light" lunch.
- You suffer from high blood pressure because you are dissatisfied with your lot in life—family, job and social life.
- You want to stop taking Valium because you think it makes you "spacy" but your doctor feels that it's helping you.

- You would like to meditate or offer a prayer at a restaurant, but are afraid people will stare at you when your head is bowed.
- You avoid talking to someone, yet you realize that a few words would open up a new relationship.
- You have a difficult time introducing yourself to someone who intrigues and fascinates you.
- You don't want to drink alcoholic beverages but find it extremely difficult and embarrassing to say "No thank you, I don't drink."

Immobilization, as far as I'm concerned, is a great energy waster. You will live a more energetic life if you break away from this pattern of inaction and begin to attack the things that bother you.

Once you understand that personal energy is your job, examine yourself before starting any program of improvement. That's one of my many complaints regarding all the popular diets. They rush you headlong into a crash program of all this and none of that, without assessing your nutritional needs. You may find that poor nutrition is the key to your energy problem. Or your problem may be stress. Possibly it's obesity. Quite probably, it's a combination. Zero in on the one area that concerns you most. Then begin your trek to more energy by working on that problem.

Avoid the pitfall of trying to change all your behavior at once. People who try to give up smoking and coffee at the same time, and then start exercising as well, usually are not successful. When you have experienced success in one area and feel good about what you have done, then move on to another area of concern. There's nothing like some success to bring on more success.

I have a good friend who every New Year's Eve resolved to give up smoking, cut back on his coffee, start exercising, and lose 15 pounds. He was filled with excellent intentions, but the change was too dramatic.

This past year I convinced him to pick one area and get that under control. I told him to focus on positive things such as exercise, not on his negative addictions of smoking and drugs. It's my position that negative addictions will disappear when positive addictions become commonplace.

My friend decided to spend 30 minutes a day walking. By mid-July he was jogging two to three miles every other day. At the end of the summer, he came to me and said, "I've dropped about seven pounds, even though I didn't pay attention to my diet, and have continued to exercise. Now, I think I'm ready to cut back on my coffee."

I think my friend's approach is best. Trying to do everything at once is counterproductive.

A Lifelong Process

Building energy is a lifelong process. Make changes when you are good and ready for them. The process is evolutionary, and dynamic as well. You make commitments, evaluate those changes, and then decide to keep, change, or modify as you experience new energy-building techniques. It's a maturation process. You come to an understanding of your body, mind, and spirit. And that takes time. Don't try to do everything at once. It won't work.

The simple checklist in Table 6-1 may help you define the area you should work on and where you'll probably have the greatest success and then be able to move on. This checklist will give you an idea of what areas you are doing well in and the areas in which you feel you need help. It will help crystallize your maximum personal energy goals and program.

Once you have identified your major area of concern, follow the principles outlined in the respective section of Section III.

Your Self-Assessment

Look over Table 6-1. After a brief introduction, you'll find six statements. Read each one carefully, then circle a number on the left that best describes your level of achievement. Be truthful, yet fair. Then, check the box on the right that indicates your level of satisfaction. Again, be honest. If you scored poorly in a given area, yet you really are satisfied to stay at that level, admit it. No one has to know what you think of yourself—except you.

Checklist Review

Now go over your responses on the right and pinpoint those areas where you feel you need improvement. That's where you need to start in your quest for more energy. Maybe you even want to turn ahead to a chapter that deals with an area that you feel is most urgent. That's fine. You're the boss. Regardless, you're the only one that can get the ball rolling. Just do me a favor and attack the problem systematically.

Planning for Energy

To begin, have a plan of action rather than trying to do everything at once. The following steps may help you.

Admit Your Problem

Unless you admit you have a problem, you will never solve it. Table 6-1 is a good place to start. The right-hand column labeled "Level of Satisfaction" is the most important part of that survey. You may score yourself rather low in the area of making and maintaining friendships, but as far as you're concerned, that's just fine with you. You see no reason for improvement. Your neighbor might perceive it to be a problem. Your husband may perceive it to be a problem. I might perceive it to be a problem. But if it doesn't bother you, there is no sense in trying to change it. You must *admit* that you are too fat, eat poorly, don't get along well with others, or whatever, before you can correct any of these areas. Once you have selected an area you can comfortably admit is a problem, you're ready for the next step.

Decide to Change

How many times have you heard one of your smoking friends declare, "One of these days I've got to quit smoking these things."? That's the way we think when it comes to doing something about our energy problem. We placate ourselves by thinking that all we need to do is go on a crash diet, start to jog, try to get to bed earlier, or take time to learn a hobby or read a book. As you know, it just doesn't happen that way. You need to make a conscious decision that you want to do something about your energy level.

Take Stock of Your Condition

The survey gave you a general idea of what problem areas may contribute to your lack of energy. Once you have selected an area that you can admit presents a problem, and have decided to do something about that problem, be specific and evaluate your problem. For example, let's say that you are not satisfied with the way you eat. You select Item #3 under "Eating Well" as an area that needs improvement because you do not take time to relax and enjoy your meals, and instead eat your food on the run or in front of the television. You would like to do something about that.

Taking stock of that problem involves a closer look at mealtime. Why don't you take the time to relax and enjoy meals? What causes you to hurry? How much time is actually spent at the meal table? What sort of activities are taking place while you are eating? Answering these questions will help you to pinpoint the reason why this has become a problem in your particular life space.

Planning the Attack, Getting Started, and Sticking to It

Just doing something about your energy problem will probably be an energy lift, but you probably have a huge list of excuses that inhibits you. I suppose I could fill a book with the excuses people have given for not doing something about their energy level. Yet as far as I'm concerned, there's only one valid excuse for a slave to a lack of energy: "I choose not to do anything about it."

If you really want to do something, you will find a way to do it. In short, you choose to do it. Approach energy in the same way. If you choose to live an energetic life, you will. The sooner you get started incorporating your plan, the sooner you will start seeing the results.

My suggestion now is to read each of the following sections. Don't skim over any unless you now know *exactly* what you want to change in your life. After you've completed reading this book, take the test in Table 6-1 again. It's possible that new information has changed your opinion on what area you really need to emphasize. After completing this reevaluation, read the pertinent chapter again carefully. Then review the goal-setting chapter and get going. When you achieve a desirable level, move on to a new area of concern.

Once you begin to see some progress, no one will stop you—they won't have the energy.

Table 6-1.   Maximum Personal Energy Self Test

Enjoying Life

Enjoyment and energy are like strawberries and cream. They complement each other. If your daily routine has degenerated into mere existence, perhaps you need to evaluate your own attitudes and expectations. Sometimes we get out of life just what we expect. How about you?*

LEVEL OF ACHIEVEMENT	ENJOYING LIFE	LEVEL OF SATISFACTION		
Low High	SELF-ASSESSMENT	OK	NEEDS IMPROVEMENT	COULD BE IMPROVED BUT NOT A CONCERN AT THIS TIME
1 2 3 4 5	(1) I like to find time to be quiet and relax.	❏	❏	❏
1 2 3 4 5	(2) I like to express myself in art, music, dance, sports, and hobbies.	❏	❏	❏
1 2 3 4 5	(3) I can accept all of my feelings such as being mad, sad, glad, and frightened.	❏	❏	❏
1 2 3 4 5	(4) I am often happy, and I find it easy to laugh	❏	❏	❏
1 2 3 4 5	(5) When I make mistakes I admit them and learn from them.	❏	❏	❏
1 2 3 4 5	(6) I can tell when I am reacting to stress and have a plan for reducing that stress.	❏	❏	❏

*SOURCE: Based on some of the work done by Robert Allen, Ph.D., and the Frost Valley YMCA staff.

Table 6-1.   Maximum Personal Energy Self Test

Enjoying Exercise

Becoming physically fit is a tremendous boost to energy. The person who is fit can work eight hours at the office and still have plenty of "go" left over to enjoy an active life at home, in the garden, on the golf course, or with a hobby. Just how do you rate?

LEVEL OF ACHIEVEMENT		ENJOYING EXERCISE	LEVEL OF SATISFACTION		
Low	High	SELF-ASSESSMENT	OK	NEEDS IMPROVEMENT	COULD BE IMPROVED BUT NOT A CONCERN AT THIS TIME
1 2 3 4 5		(1) I bike, swim, run, or walk for at least 30 minutes, 3 or more times a week.	❏	❏	❏
1 2 3 4 5		(2) Whenever possible, I walk or ride a bike instead of using cars, elevators, escalators, etc.	❏	❏	❏
1 2 3 4 5		(3) I do some form of stretching several times per week.	❏	❏	❏
1 2 3 4 5		(4) I participate in sports for reasons other than competition.	❏	❏	❏
1 2 3 4 5		(5) It is fun for me to be physically active.	❏	❏	❏
1 2 3 4 5		(6) I try to learn one new sport every two years.	❏	❏	❏

Table 6-1.   Maximum Personal Energy Self Test

Eating Well

An engine needs a steady supply of good, clean fuel in order to run efficiently. So do you. Food provides that fuel, and like the engine, your body needs a regular supply of good, nutritious food. Too much of this or too little of that will drain your energy supply. Is that something you need to work on?

LEVEL OF ACHIEVEMENT		EATING WELL	LEVEL OF SATISFACTION		
LOW	HIGH	SELF-ASSESSMENT	OK	NEEDS IMPROVEMENT	COULD BE IMPROVED BUT NOT A CONCERN AT THIS TIME
1 2 3 4 5		(1) I eat a balanced diet and enjoy a variety of fresh, natural foods.	❏	❏	❏
1 2 3 4 5		(2) I try to eat foods with little added sugar, salt, and/or saturated fat.	❏	❏	❏
1 2 3 4 5		(3) I take time to relax and enjoy my meals. I also eat my food in one location (at a table).	❏	❏	❏
1 2 3 4 5		(4) I consume very little coffee, colas, or other foods high in caffeine.	❏	❏	❏
1 2 3 4 5		(5) I eat three well-balanced meals a day—breakfast, lunch, and dinner.	❏	❏	❏
1 2 3 4 5		(6) My diet contains a relatively low amount of fat (30 percent or less), a moderate to low amount of meat, and regular portions of complex carbohydrates.	❏	❏	❏

Table 6-1. Maximum Personal Energy Self Test

Staying Slim

Staying slim involves a balance between your physical activity and eating behaviors. To have a low percentage of fat and your weight under control, you must select big muscle activities such as walking, running, bicycling, and swimming. You should also build extra activities into your day. That is, never lie down when you can sit, never sit when you can stand, never stand when you can walk. These physical activities should also be complemented with good eating practices.

LEVEL OF ACHIEVEMENT		STAYING SLIM	LEVEL OF SATISFACTION		
Low	High	SELF-ASSESSMENT	OK	NEEDS IMPROVEMENT	COULD BE IMPROVED BUT NOT A CONCERN AT THIS TIME
1 2 3 4 5		(1) I bike, swim, run, or walk for at least 30 minutes, three or more times a week.	❏	❏	❏
1 2 3 4 5		(2) Whenever possible, I walk or ride a bike instead of using cars, elevators, escalators, etc.	❏	❏	❏
1 2 3 4 5		(3) I eat foods high in nutrients and low in calories.	❏	❏	❏
1 2 3 4 5		(4) I eat three meals a day— breakfast, lunch, and dinner.	❏	❏	❏
1 2 3 4 5		(5) I don't eat when I'm bored or under pressure.	❏	❏	❏
1 2 3 4 5		(6) I cannot pinch more than an inch of fat on my body.	❏	❏	❏

Table 6-1. Maximum Personal Energy Self Test

Relating to Others

A few years ago, it wasn't unusual to hear someone say, "Boy, she really gets me down!" That was a good description of how poor relationships can physically sap your strength. Nobody likes to fight or argue. The effects on energy are total: emotional and physical energy is lost. How well do you relate?

LEVEL OF ACHIEVEMENT		RELATING TO OTHERS	LEVEL OF SATISFACTION		
Low	High	Self-Assessment	OK	Needs Improvement	Could be Improved But Not a Concern at This Time
1 2 3 4 5		(1) I enjoy my family and get along well with my family members.	❑	❑	❑
1 2 3 4 5		(2) I can make and maintain friendships.	❑	❑	❑
1 2 3 4 5		(3) I try to listen to others without always thinking of what I want to say.	❑	❑	❑
1 2 3 4 5		(4) I would rather talk to someone about how I feel than keep it inside.	❑	❑	❑
1 2 3 4 5		(5) I am open to people who are different than I (age, race, religion and interests).	❑	❑	❑
1 2 3 4 5		(6) I am able to give and receive love.	❑	❑	❑

Table 6-1. Maximum Personal Energy Self Test

Taking Care of Yourself

There are many kings of things we can do in an effort to get energy. We smoke, do drugs, abuse alcohol, take unnecessary risks, and watch violence and mayhem for stimulation. These activities put the emphasis on something outside of you for a lift. These are negative addictions, as Dr. William Glasser, author of *Positive Addiction*, calls them. Ultimately they can drag you down.

Below is a checklist to see how you're doing on these behaviors. But there is one radical difference—you will not find a corresponding section in Section III on Taking Care Of Yourself. I do not tell you how to stop these behaviors. That's because I know that if you opt for the other positive addictions listed in the book—learning how to enjoy life, participating in aerobic exercise, eating good food, staying slim, and relating well to others—there will be no need for your negative addictions. I want you to emphasize the positive.

LEVEL OF ACHIEVEMENT		TAKING CARE OF YOURSELF	LEVEL OF SATISFACTION		
Low	High	SELF-ASSESSMENT	OK	NEEDS IMPROVEMENT	COULD BE IMPROVED BUT NOT A CONCERN AT THIS TIME
1 2 3 4 5		(1) I do not smoke cigarettes.	❑	❑	❑
1 2 3 4 5		(2) I *rarely* (not more than once every 2 months) take self-prescribed medicine, i.e., aspirin-type products, suppositories, and other over-the-counter drugs.	❑	❑	❑
1 2 3 4 5		(3) I drink 1 to 2 ounces of alcohol or less daily.	❑	❑	❑
1 2 3 4 5		(4) I make up my own mind about drug and alcohol use, despite what others are doing.	❑	❑	❑
1 2 3 4 5		(5) I ask my physician on the necessity of my taking medication prescribed for me.	❑	❑	❑
1 2 3 4 5		(6) I find I am not dependent on external stimuli (drugs, alcohol, cigarettes, sugar, and thrill activities) to get me high.	❑	❑	❑

►►►Section III:►►►
Mastery of Skills

▶▶ *Enjoying Life* ▶ ▶ ▶ ▶ ▶ ▶

Fighting Back

You've learned that not handling stress properly can ruin your maximum personal energy. You've also learned that you can fight back—if you want to. But to do it you need skills and strategies that work.

For years, psychologists have used the term "coping" to demonstrate an ability to survive and handle today's pressures and changes. While the term is good, Dr. Wayne Dyer has convinced me that a better term is "mastery". Coping implies just getting by. Mastery implies that you're in charge. I like that. Therefore, I want to give you some mastery skills that you can use to enjoy life to its fullest.

Scheduling Time

The ability to effectively schedule your time is an important skill in preventing stress from depleting your supply of energy. In fact, you may have read previous suggestions from other authors and complained, "Good things to do, but I just don't have the time or energy to do them." Usually that's because many people have not assumed control over the day. Instead, they literally run through a busy list of things to do, try to do them all at once, and hope to someday get "a little room to breathe." Life is busy for everyone. Yet the ones who always seem to have room to breathe are the ones who have learned to manage their time efficiently.

Basically, you need to look at your day in terms of four areas: work, sleep, relaxation, and family and social obligations. Obviously, your working segment is pretty much determined for you. That is, work takes up approximately eight hours of each weekday.

Write down a schedule for work and try to follow it, making a point of doing the most important or difficult things first. Make small decisions promptly—in most matters any decision is better than no decision. Use all the help available to you, delegating work when it is more efficient to do so, and say no when others are in a position to do a piece of work more efficiently and effectively than you.

Alan Lakein suggests listing top goals for both the short term (six months) and long term (lifetime), then listing activities that will take you toward these goals. The idea is to put an A, B, or C next to each according to its importance (if the list is long, A_1, A_2, A_3, etc., may be used). An A activity (or part of one, starting with the easiest or most important task) should be done first each day, preferably early in the day, to be followed by B's, and if time permits, by Cs. A new list of priorities can be drawn up at the beginning or end of each day to reflect changes in emphasis. The A goals for the week ahead can be prepared on Friday afternoon. Lifetime goals, based on the day-to-day and weekly goals, can be mapped at longer intervals. Time each day can be set aside to get in at least one A_1 task for one or more long-range goal.

For overwhelmed people who worry about never getting to their C tasks, Lakein cites what he calls the 80/20 rule. "If all items are arranged in order of value, 80 percent of the value would come from only 20 percent of the items, while the remaining 20 percent of the value would come from 80 percent of the items." Lakein therefore urges his clients to avoid the tendency to do C tasks, which are usually simpler and therefore more tempting than the vital As. The Cs are relatively insignificant anyway and if they are postponed, the need to do some of them may disappear as time passes.

Making Your Time Strategy Work

There are a number of ways this strategy can be implemented. I use what I call the "three-drawer concept." In my office desk there are three drawers. My A tasks go in the top drawer, my B tasks go in the middle drawer, and my C tasks go in the bottom drawer. If I had a fourth drawer it would be a waste basket.

Another Lakein suggestion is to sort through goals originally classified as B's and reclassify them as As or Cs—especially C's. These can be kept in a file folder in a drawer and reviewed periodically for action or disposal. At first reading, incoming mail can be sorted into folders labeled Action, Information, and Deferred and given appropriate priority on the daily list.

As an added help in becoming more efficient, those using the Lakein approach are urged to frequently ask themselves "Lakein's Question"— "What is the best use of my time right now?"

The next area, sleep, may need some special attention. Since a proper amount of sleep is pivotal to abundant energy, you may need to adjust your daily schedule so that you get to bed on time. For most people, six hours of sleep is an absolute minimum. Your own demands may be higher. If so, don't ignore those demands. You will get more done in a shorter period of time if your body is sufficiently rested.

So if you spend eight hours at work, and seven hours sleeping, that leaves nine hours for fun and games, right? Of course not. You've got to mow the lawn, repair the leaky faucet, go shopping, take the kids to the dentist, pay the bills, and everything else. But you do not have to do all of these things at once.

Follow Lakein's advice again or try this: make a list of all those social and household obligations that aren't connected with your job, but must be done. Beside each one, put an approximate amount of your time it takes to do the tasks. Now underline those that could be omitted. Using this list as a guide, make a schedule for each day of the week, setting aside a time for each of the "absolute activities." If there are not enough hours in the week to get everything done, cross out the ones that are followed with question marks. Make sure you include time for relaxation and enjoyment. Then, tape the schedule in a place where you'll see it often, and follow it rigidly for one week. I think you'll find that it works. Why? Because being in control gives a tremendous sense of satisfaction and accomplishment. That is a great ally in your battle for more energy.

Positive Mental Outlook

David Fink, M.D., a psychiatrist who has done extensive work in the area of stress and nervous tension, refers to the "play spirit" of a man or woman. In counseling his patients who are troubled, he encourages them to take the play spirit into everything they do. That is, approach each activity as if it were going to be playful and fun. While that may sound simplistic, the concept is important. The attitude with which we approach a situation often dictates how that situation affects us. If you go to work with a feeling of dread or boredom, the chances are you'll get just that.

So my first recommendation is to change your outlook. When you get up in the morning, tell yourself, "Today is going to be a great day!" Approach each task that faces you in a new light. Look for things that are amusing. Try to avoid negative thoughts by replacing them with positive ones. I know it doesn't always work this way. But you'd be surprised how a more positive approach to a wearisome situation can turn the experience into a pleasant one.

Getting into the play spirit will help, but obviously it's only the beginning. After all, you need a little play occasionally to keep that positive attitude. According to Fink, play is anything you do that you can drop as soon as it ceases to amuse. Something you can take or leave alone. Consequently, some of the things you once thought were play are now drudgery. Bowling leagues, coffee klatches, bridge nights, and even jogging, began with play in mind, but may have turned into an obligation you can't or won't give up. You'd like to quit the softball team, but the teammates are counting on you. You have to attend the neighborhood study group because, well, it's expected of you. Soon, play has become work.

To remedy that, look for new ways to play. Usually that means returning to basic, simple activities, perhaps even activities that seem childish. For starters, a hobby or special project can be play. Hobbies are often abandoned by adults when they board the work/family bandwagon. Interestingly, that's when stress usually begins to become a problem. If you collected stamps in the sixth grade, dig out your old collection—it may rekindle interest and give you something to play with. If that doesn't suit you, try something on the creative side. Learn to dance. Grab a brush, canvas, and palette, and give painting a try. Or learn to play a musical instrument. The goal is not to become a world master but to divert your attention from the doldrums while having a little fun.

Expression of Feelings and Emotional Awareness

Emotional health and a zest for living are impossible unless we acknowledge our feelings, express them appropriately, and use them effectively. Unfortunately, our culture does not respect emotions, and we are taught to hide, deny, or repress our feelings lest we "lose control" and "act irrationally."

This is particularly true in the business world, where the direct expression of feelings is usually discouraged, and where the ability to deal with feelings is much less valued than the capacity to handle ideas. Nevertheless, as behavioral scientists have noted, many of the most desirable traits in business—as well as personal life—are derived from emotions. These valuable qualities include creativity, motivation, loyalty, enthusiasm, and cooperation.

When feelings are stifled—whether at home or on the job—the person harboring "unacceptable" emotions cannot function fully and freely, for precious energy must be wasted to maintain an unauthentic self, to create an "image," and to "play the game." Furthermore, if feelings are not shared and dealt with face-to-face, problems that have been "solved" by rational means don't stay solved for long—the underlying emotional conflict simply translates itself into other terms, erupting sooner or later into another crisis at work or home.

On the other hand, experimental evidence suggests that if a person is allowed to express negative feelings to the individual who has aroused them, he or she will feel friendlier later than if the bad feelings are forced to remain "underground." If the expression of anger, anxiety, or frustration is not met with a counterattack or with an immediate attempt to introduce rationality, but is encouraged by the listener and received with understanding and acceptance ("You seem upset. What's troubling you?..." "I think I know how you feel."), then the upset person will be able to work through the negative feeling and arrive at a more objective assessment of the situation. The point is that "feelings press for discharge," and when they are denied they can become a barrier to closeness with others and to working rationally and harmoniously toward common goals.

Handling Problems

Dealing with problems isn't peripheral to life, it's the essence of it, for whether we realize it or not, most human behavior consists of problem solving. Those who have the most success at understanding and solving problems independently or with the help of others have been found to share one characteristic: considerable confidence in and esteem for themselves and others. This kind of positive, facilitating attitude toward dealing with problems can be developed by jettisoning useless emotions, such as guilt, which shackles us to the past, or worry, which projects us into the imagined future. As psychologist Wayne Dyer has noted, neither of these all-too-common feelings changes anything; they can only rob us of the confidence and self-esteem we sorely need to tackle the problem and—equally harmful—distract us from the problem while siphoning off energy that should be directed into purposeful action.

Another tendency that undermines our ability to deal with problems is blaming. When we spend time and energy cursing fate or railing against people, circumstances, or even ourselves, we are simply expressing frustration. We are not correcting the problem. Indeed, by indulging in blame we are persuading ourselves that we are passive victims incapable of righting what's wrong.

Guilt, worry, blame, and fear all promote procrastination, and are most likely to do so when we are confronted by a problem. To fight the tendency to avoid problems by taking refuge in delay, time management consultant Alan Lakein suggests strategies such as structuring your time and the things around you so you can't use your favorite escape routes. Possibility thinking Robert Schuller's technique is to make a habit of asking yourself, "What is my biggest problem and what have I done about it today?" Another approach to handling procrastination linked to stress is to train yourself to be more of a stress-seeker and to view problems as challenges.

Studies performed by Susan C. Kobasa and Salvatore R. Maddi, both psychologists at the University of Chicago, indicate that stress can be a positive element for some people. They contend that stress-resistant people have a specific set of attitudes toward life that make up what is known as a "hardy personality." Those attitudes are an openness to change, a feeling of involvement in whatever they are doing, and a sense of control over events! One of the studies showed that people who rated high in these attitudes had fewer stress-related illnesses than others. On the other hand, those who rated low in "hardiness" avoided their problems—distracting themselves by watching more TV, drinking too much, taking tranquilizers, and sleeping more. Instead of solving problems, they ignored them.

Steps in problem-solving as articulated by one successful executive are (1) to identify the problem, (2) to find the causes by investigation (that is, by talking to all involved and asking Who-What-Where-How-and-When questions, then making comparisons and deductions), (3) to weigh the possible inferences, and (4) to decide on the best solution, which should be economical, efficient, fair, based on facts, and meet current needs but also anticipate future needs.

Self-Actualization

As human beings, we have a hierarchy of needs that must be met if we are to continue to live and to evolve as individuals. Our most basic need is the physiological one for food, air, and water, and this will motivate us sufficiently in life-or-death situations, as will the next highest need, which is for security (protection from physical harm). As these requirements are met, we continue up the ladder, first seeking the fulfillment of social, or affiliative, needs, which represent the longing for acceptance by others, then striving to meet esteem, or ego needs, which involve recognition by others. At the very top of the hierarchy of needs most social scientists place self-actualization (sometimes called self-fulfillment). This has been variously defined as becoming one's best self, achieving self-recognition, making the decision to take responsibility for self-motivation, realizing one's potential, and continuing to grow and be creative.

The behavior characterizing self-actualizing people stands in sharp contrast to the self-destructive activities engaged in by those who have not been able to satisfy and transcend their more basic needs. Through interviews with selected subjects, psychologist Abraham Maslow found self-actualizers to be totally unique in the expression of their varied selves, yet alike in being authentic, involved in a cause outside themselves that makes the work-joy dichotomy disappear, and in devoting their lives to a search for ultimate values with which they identify themselves, such as truth, goodness, beauty, justice, order, aliveness, and playfulness.

I would like to emphasize these latter points. All too often people seek to be self-actualized. In so doing, they turn in on themselves and become self-centered. Truthfully, a person "finds" him or herself by "losing" him or herself. That is, he or she gives of themself to another cause, person or institution without an expected return. This is self-fulfillment.

Maslow claims all of us have the impulse toward self-fulfillment, but most of us never make it because we fear our highest possibilities—a fact revealed by our mixed feelings toward great people. Society itself may be encouraging us to remain inhibited and self-divided.

Our task, then, is to give up only as much as we must to routine and tedium and to strike out on a unique path of lifelong learning which may, as Buckminster Fuller has suggested, involved the "self-administered unlearning of most of what we've been taught in school." We can hasten our progress toward self-actualization by (1) allowing ourselves to experience life fully, without self-consciousness or self-awareness, (2) making choices based on growth (progression) rather than fear (regression), (3) listening to our inner totality—The Self, (4) being honest when we are in doubt, (5) preparing ourselves to do well what we want to do, (6) seeking and surrendering to peak experiences, in which we transcend ourselves and experience moments of self-realization, (7) recognizing that we are the by-product of many people who have gone before us, and that our values, belief systems, education and our station in life are the result of many people who have sacrificed for us, and (8) identifying our defenses and finding the courage to give them up and to invest the people, events, and objects around us with symbolic and eternal value. Much of this is a payback, if you will, to those who helped make us who we are.

Becoming Less Vulnerable

It's not going to be easy, this business of fighting back from a lifestyle based on almost total vulnerability to stress. There will be setbacks along the way, apparent failures. At times, you will be tempted to give up. I know that I face times like that occasionally, and usually they occur just when I think I've got things under control. So I'd like to share some thoughts with you that have helped me deal with those setbacks. I would like to claim them as my own kernels of truth, but the credit goes to Hans Selye:

1. Regardless of how much you want to be loved, it's useless to try to befriend someone who continuously rejects you.

2. Face the fact that there is no such thing as perfection. Your highest goal is to be the best you can be.

3. Returning to a more simple lifestyle can add more pleasure to life than all that wealth and extravagance you've been struggling to obtain.

4. Before you waste a lot of energy trying to fight your way out of a situation, ask yourself if it's really worth fighting for.

5. Focus only on what is pleasant in your life, forgetting anything painful or ugly.

6. When you face your most difficult hour, try to recall and dwell on a past success. A sense of frustration can totally immobilize you. You can avoid that by concentrating on even the slightest bright spot in your past.

7. Never try to detour from unpleasant tasks. Face them as soon as possible so that you can move on to more enjoyable things.

8. There are no pat answers or special formulas for success that will fit everyone. Choose from a wide variety of advice only those things that fit your own unique personality.

If you follow the suggestions in this chapter, you will not eliminate stress from your life. Stress is here to stay. However, applying these ideas to your life wherever they are relevant and possible will bring you a long way toward dealing with the stress that has sapped so much of your energy.

The Three Rs

By now you have an idea of what stress is doing to your energy levels. You also have some idea of how to deal with them. Here I want to give you some important extra helps—the three Rs: Relaxation, Recreation, and Rest. It is important to note that I use recreation in the true sense of the word: activities that recreate with a sense of newness and vitality.

You can't run from stress. I'm convinced that one reason so many people do not enjoy life is that they expend too much energy running from it, trying to avoid it. In this chapter you will discover some techniques and responses to stress that enable you to really live rather than merely exist.

Relaxation and Recreation: Their True Value

Such utility aside, the development of impersonal interests is important, if only because favorite physical or mental pursuits can provide a resource and a respite at times when our central concerns in life are going badly.

But how do these friendly, impersonal interests get translated into true pleasure—that is, into the kind that is restorative? Drama critic Walter Kerr suggests the more we want or expect to have a good time, the less likely we are to have one—a phenomenon that applies to social events, sexual experiences, everything. It is necessary, says Kerr, to "quiet the will to please the mind"—to hold the self in abeyance and cultivate "a relaxed grip," a state of readiness that is not acquisitive. The paradox is that only by bringing ourselves to a willingness to let go can we firmly grasp the pleasure we so desire. The problem, Kerr maintains, is that "as twentieth-century adults we have become compulsive users," and have lost the ability to contemplate experiences, things, and people—that is, to view them attentively in an appreciative and relaxed, but nonacquisitive way. A direct contradiction to the way most Americans live.

Contemplation and the restorative pleasure it makes possible are also being threatened by the frantic pace of modern life, which keeps us so busy and distracted that we don't have time to contemplate even fragments of our experience, let alone the whole of our lives. The way back to this profound kind of recreation seems to lie in undoing the conditioning that our industrialized society has imposed on us—we must once again learn to value doing things, instead of getting them, and the insights that we can create for ourselves rather than the things and experiences we can buy.

Relaxation

People often misinterpret what type of "rest" their bodies need. After a grueling day at the office you reward yourself by flopping down on the couch to rest and recover from a stress-filled day, when what your body really might need is physical activity. Or, you pour yourself a drink when a chat with your spouse would be better for both of you. As you will see from some of the stress management techniques discussed in this chapter, you need to reassess traditional methods of relaxing, i.e., sleep, rest, watching TV. Often, those only postpone the problem.

The first group of techniques here confront your stress via relaxation. Not all of them will work for you, but try each exercise at least once before you pass judgment. Think of this section as a catalogue of techniques available for you. Some you may not need. Some may not work for you, yet do wonders for the other guy. By becoming familiar with each of them you will be better equipped to turn stress into energy.

Body Scanning

This may sound exotic, but it isn't. It's a simple technique to become more aware of your body. Lie down on the floor and close your eyes. Starting with your toes, think your way up your body asking yourself, "Where do I feel tension?" If you discover your jaw muscles are tight, exaggerate them slightly by tightening them more. Remind yourself that this takes effort and if continued over a long period of time you will become exhausted. Then relax those muscles and move on to the next source of tension. This activity need not take more than five minutes. Try doing it just before you leave for work and again before going to bed.

Progressive Relaxation

This technique, and a book by the same name, was developed by Dr. Edmund Jacobson in the early 1900's. It is based on the premise that the body responds to anxiety-provoking thoughts with muscle tension and that deep muscle relaxation counters the effects of that tension.

Repeat the following procedures at least once, tensing each muscle group from 5 to 7 seconds and then relaxing from 20 to 30 seconds. Focus on the contrast between the sensations of tension and relaxation.

1. Curl both fists, tightening biceps and forearms. Relax.
2. Wrinkle up forehead. At the same time, press your head as far back as possible, roll it clockwise in a complete circle. Reverse. Now wrinkle up the muscles in your face by frowning, squinting, pursing your lips, pressing your tongue against the roof of your mouth, and hunching your shoulders. Relax.
3. Arch back as you take a deep breath into the chest. Hold. Relax. Take a deep breath, pressing out the stomach. Hold. Relax.
4. Pull feet and toes back toward face, tightening shins. Hold. Relax. Curl toes while simultaneously tightening calves, thighs, and buttocks. Hold. Relax.

Make sure in the relaxation stage the muscle group is totally relaxed. When you think the muscles are completely relaxed, tell yourself to relax just a little bit more. Also, don't overly tighten the muscles when you are tensing, as it could cause a cramp.

This technique will take some practice at first. Eventually, however, it will be possible to relax your entire body in just a few moments. It's a great one for desk-sitters and can be performed almost anywhere.

Meditation

Meditation may take many forms, but regardless of how you meditate, it affects your body and mind and gives you energy in many different ways. Meditators state that 20 minutes of their activity is equivalent to the boost you expect to receive from a cup or two of coffee. Scientists tell us that the reason for this lift is that meditation causes a significant drop in metabolism. This drop is similar to several hours of sleeping—yet in meditation the drop is achieved in a matter of minutes. Heart rate and breathing also slow down while anxiety decreases.

Research also suggests that meditators learn how to handle their stress better. A study reported in the February 1976 issue of Psychology Today in the article, *Meditation Helps Break the Stress Spiral,* by David Golman, illustrates this point. The experimenters selected two groups of people to watch a highly stressful film—accidents in a woodworking shop. One group consisted of experienced meditators while the other group of people wanted to learn meditation but had not yet tried it.

The researchers divided these people into two subgroups. Twenty minutes before the showing of the film the meditating people were told to either meditate or simply relax. One-half of the meditators relaxed for 20 minutes and the other half of the meditators meditated for 20 minutes. The other group of subjects was split in a similar manner. The first group was told to relax while the second group was taught a meditation technique in 20 minutes.

The results of the study were revealing. Those who had meditated (experienced and inexperienced) had more signs of alarm just before an accident occurred on the screen. They had higher heart rates, more sweating, and so forth. Interestingly, they returned to normal more quickly afterwards, which indicates that their bodies were handling the stress quite well. The response to stress was true of all meditators—the novices included. Even the meditators who relaxed responded similarly. The researchers came to the inescapable conclusion that meditation apparently had immediate and long-term effects on the body. It had long-term effects since the experienced meditators who simply relaxed also handled the stressful viewing quite well. Meditation helps people cope better with stress.

Relaxation Response

Relaxation Response is a technique set forth by Dr. Herbert Benson, a Harvard cardiologist. After studying various ways of relaxing he found that meditation, yoga, praying, and similar kinds of activities elicited relaxation on the part of the participant and were probably energizing. Benson outlines a simple way of soothing your body during stress. He suggests that you engage in the following Relaxation Response type of activity twice a day—early morning and in the evening. Begin your daily "de-stressing" with these suggestions:

1. Sit quietly in a comfortable position.
2. Close your eyes.
3. Deeply relax all your muscles, beginning at your feet and progressing up to your face. Keep them relaxed.
4. Breathe through your nose. Become aware of your breathing. As you breathe out say the word, "ONE," silently to yourself. For example, breathe IN...OUT, "ONE"; IN...OUT, "ONE"; and so on. Breathe easily and naturally.

5. Continue for 10 to 20 minutes. You may open your eyes to check the time, but do not use an alarm. When you finish, sit quietly for several minutes, at first with your eyes closed and later with your eyes open. For a few minutes, do not stand up.

6. Do not worry about whether you are successful in achieving a deep level of relaxation. Maintain a passive attitude and permit relaxation to occur at its own pace. While distracting thoughts occur, try to ignore them by not dwelling upon them and return to repeating "ONE." With practice, the response should come with little effort. Practice the technique once or twice daily, but not within two hours after any meal, since the digestive processes seem to interfere with the elicitation of the Relaxation Response.

Imagining

As a youngster, you probably escaped the boredom of numerous situations by turning on your imaginative powers. Oftentimes, you left the stifling lecture period and joined King Arthur at the Round Table. By occasionally engaging in this same activity, you can treat yourself to some bright spots in what might be a stress-filled day.

There are no special rules to follow when you use your imagination to create relaxation and relief from stress. Whenever you sense a tenseness invading your body, close your eyes and try to imagine something especially pleasant: wading in a cool mountain stream, walking along a mountain trail, seeing a calm, blue sky, or gliding through the air in a rope swing. Always try to imagine yourself in a distant setting, away from your daily routine.

After imagining for three to four minutes, open your eyes, change your position, stretch, and resume what you were doing. One caution: don't become a constant daydreamer. A few, brief sessions each day will give you a sense of heightened energy and emotional well-being. Spending more than five to ten minutes several times a day at this may cost you your job—thus more stress and less energy!

Breathing Exercises

Everyone knows how to breathe. Yet paying attention to different types of breathing can help restore energy lost through stress. Try the following techniques occasionally for a lift.

Deep Breathing

Lie down on the floor with your knees slightly bent, one hand on your abdomen, the other on your chest. Inhale deeply through your nose, trying to control your breathing with your abdomen. Your chest should move only a little. Smile slightly, exhaling through your mouth, making a quiet, relaxing sound like the wind as you gently release your breath. Continue for three to ten minutes.

Sighing

Sighs and yawns are signs that your body needs more energy-rich oxygen. A sigh provides you with a rush of air and helps to reduce tension. Simply take a deep breath and sigh deeply, letting out a sound of relief as the air leaves your lungs. Don't rush it out and don't think about inhaling. Just let the air come in naturally. Repeat this six to eight times whenever you feel the need for it.

The Windmill Breath

Stand up with your arms stretched out at your sides. Take a deep breath and as you exhale slowly, swing your arms alternately like a windmill. Repeat two or three times. This is especially helpful if you have been bent over your work for several hours and are feeling tense. You will return to your work feeling more alert and alive.

Relaxation Throughout the Day

Program relaxing activities into your day. Choose anything that takes your mind off the hustle and bustle of everyday life and produces a pleasant feeling. Read a book, enjoy a quiet talk with your spouse, work in the garden, help one of your kids put together a model airplane, or listen to music. It is important that each day you experience this type of pleasant activity. Spending a few minutes genuinely relaxing can restore that lost energy and enable you to finish the day on an upbeat note.

Spending a few minutes with your feet elevated and a pillow under your head can be revitalizing, but don't limit yourself to that. Experiment with different activities to see what works best in taking your mind off your problems. If you work with your head all day, you may find a hobby that requires some manual skills is just the thing. If your job requires a lot of physical labor, reading, word games, writing, or learning something new might offer more relaxation for you. Find an activity that is best for you, then allow yourself time on a regular basis to enjoy that activity.

Recreation

In addition to contemplation, there are more active forms of recreation that are restorative. Most thoughtful people agree, however, that the kind of fun that renews and truly recreates us doesn't come from overstimulation. As pointed out in Chapter 5, overstimulation of any kind is exhausting and makes us "insensitive to the pleasures of ordinary living."

Just what kinds of activities meet the requirements of being restorative without being exhausting? The ones that give us more than they take away. Bertrand Russell himself favored long nature walks and ocean swims, for he believed pursuits that bring mankind into contact with the life of the Earth are profoundly satisfying and make for lasting happiness even though their intensity may be less than that "of more exciting dissipations." Noncompetitive activities such as jogging, or any other recreation meeting the criteria for a "positive addiction" (activities that build you up rather than tear you down—that are creative rather than destructive) are another route for self-renewal.

Whatever the form of recreation we choose, it is important to remember that our psychological needs must be satisfied directly, through an active effort of our own, "and not by the substitution and distraction" and oblivion provided by escapist fare such as TV, drugs, and spectator sports. Passive entertainment makes us less alive. It is not renewing, just distracting.

Below are some recreational physical activities that help to give us mastery over stress. They help build fitness, reduce tension, make us feel good about ourselves, and energize our bodies.

Running and Other Aerobic Activities

I mention running first because I think it should have high priority. It also is the activity that has had the most research conducted about it. Some physiologists and psychiatrists have begun to advocate the use of running as therapy for stress-related problems such as the blues, depression, nervous tension, and fatigue. Thaddeus Kostrubala, M.D., a California psychiatrist, requires each of his patients to run a specified time and distance several times a week. He often runs with them, conducting his counseling "on the run." If he doesn't run himself, one of his running therapists does.

John Griest, M.D., a psychiatrist operating out of the University of Wisconsin in Madison, has used running as a very important part of a therapy program with depressed patients. He found that fatigue was a common symptom of depression and that the running helped depressed individuals alleviate that "tired overall feeling."

But not all research has been done on running. Activities such as walking are just as effective. Dr. Herbert deVries, Ph.D., a noted exercise physiologist, has said that the best tranquilizer is a brisk, 15-minute walk. One of his studies demonstrated that a short walk can be as effective in treating nervous tension as a normal dosage of a tranquilizer.

Your program of physical activity may be as informal and unstructured as adding a 15-minute walk to your lunch hour. Or, it might be as vigorous as a 40-minute run every day. The following guidelines will help you use your physical activity to reduce stress-induced fatigue:

1. Choose an activity you enjoy—just because running is "in" doesn't mean you will enjoy it. Walking or using a cross-country ski exerciser is just as effective and often fits into your daily routine quite easily.

2. Think of each session as a reward rather than an obligation— sometimes the anticipation of a little exercise is part of the "magic" of reducing fatigue.

3. Don't overdo it—within ten minutes after your exercise session, you should feel refreshed and ready to resume your schedule. If you are unduly tired and physically uncomfortable for a half hour or more after exercising, you probably overexercised. Take it easy, especially in the early stages.

4. Enjoy the physical "you"—take pride in the fact that you've joined a unique group of people who use stress rather than allow themselves to be abused by it. Remind yourself, perhaps with an air of justifiable smugness, that someone else is taking a Seconal to escape while you have opted for self-discipline and control.

5. Don't worry about the clock. Exercise at a rate that seems best for you. Do not keep comparing yourself to some arbitrary standard. The best recreation is play.

Rest and Sleep

You might compare your body to a machine or engine, for it can generate power. As with other engines, it needs rest to avoid a breakdown since your body wears out a little each day. Fortunately, proper rest keeps you from disintegrating too much, for during rest your mind and body recharge themselves.

The Benefits of Sleep

Your body is in action constantly. Sometimes slow, sometimes fast, but it's always working. When you're wide awake, your body is highly stimulated. Your mind is alert. After a period of time both your body and your mind call for a rest. They tell you it's time to slow down. When that happens you start to feel tired. You become drowsy. Sleep is the only way out.

The revitalization that occurs during sleep occurs because your nervous system is no longer stimulated. Your heart rate slows down as does your breathing rate. Your body temperature and blood pressure drop. Almost everything in your body slows down. The stimuli for your five senses are reduced substantially. It is during this time that your body's "batteries" are recharged. When you awaken you should be completely refreshed, ready to go.

REM and Non-REM Sleep

Scientists say there are two kinds of sleep. One of these is called Rapid Eye Movement or REM, during which you dream vividly. The other is Non-REM, of which there are four stages.

First Stage: Here, you're just falling asleep. Your body functions are starting to slow down. But you can be awakened easily.

Second Stage: During this stage your eyes roll from side to side. Your sleep is deep. But when you awaken you do not recall having any dreams.

Third Stage: Your body really slows down in this stage. Blood pressure and pulse rates are very low, as is your temperature. Sleep is very deep and calm.

Fourth Stage: This is the period of deepest sleep. But it is brief. Nightmares and sleepwalking can occur during this stage.

After getting to the fourth stage, you then go back to stages three, two, one, and into REM sleep. During your sleep you cycle continually through these stages three to four times. As the night continues, the REM time gets longer and the Non-REM time shorter. Each occurrence of REM sleep lasts from five minutes to over an hour. For adults, about 20 percent of their sleep is REM sleep.

The amount of REM sleep is very important, because the degree of restfulness of sleep is related to the amount of REM sleep. In studies where people were awakened each time they entered REM sleep, the result was extreme tiredness and abnormal behavior.

How Much Sleep Do You Need?

Everyone needs sleep. Most young people need somewhere around 8 to 10 hours of sleep. Newborn babies may sleep as much as 20 hours or more a day. Mature adults usually find 7 hours or less is sufficient. But there are always differences between individuals. Thomas Edison is said to have slept only 3 to 4 hours a night. He did, however, have a cot in his laboratory and he catnapped whenever fatigue got the best of him.

Two other well-known catnappers of the twentieth century are Dr. Michael DeBakey, the world famous heart specialist, and the late President

John F. Kennedy. DeBakey is able to fall asleep very quickly. When traveling by air, he simply buckles himself into his seat on the plane and immediately drops into a deep sleep. President Kennedy was able to do the same thing. During a busy and pressure-packed day, he could fall asleep quickly. He would sit down, close his eyes, and fall asleep almost immediately. In five minutes he would awaken refreshed and ready to dive into the task at hand.

People like DeBakey, Kennedy, and Edison are exceptions. So are their jobs. The work world is set up on an eight-hour schedule. Most people turn in somewhere between 9:00 p.m. and midnight and arise between 5:00 and 8:00 a.m. As a result, most people get their eight hours of sleep or so in one block of time.

Regardless, a proper amount of sleep is very important for everyone. But each person's requirements for sleep will vary. Some may need nine hours of sleep, some feel seven is enough. The key to understanding whether you are getting enough is that you should awaken spontaneously and refreshed.

Insomnia

All people at one time or another have difficulty sleeping. Some people fall asleep rather quickly but awaken in the middle of the night. Some sleepwalk or talk in their sleep. The extent to which these disorders are serious depends upon how frequently they occur. The disorders are serious if they are disturbing to the sleeper or, I should say, nonsleeper.

Insomnia, however, is the inability to sleep. One out of every 20 people reacts this way. The problem is vicious. When a person goes to bed, tosses and turns and cannot sleep, he worries. He worries because he's not getting enough sleep so he stays awake even longer—sometimes the entire night. The next night when he falls into bed he's exhausted. But he's worried. Last night he didn't get enough sleep. So he worries about this and consequently loses even more sleep. The cycle progresses in this manner: worry, less sleep, more worry, less sleep, and so on. Worrying about the insomnia only makes matters worse.

To help themselves, some people use tranquilizers and barbiturates. But these drugs interfere with normal sleep patterns. However, there are ways of getting the rest you need without resorting to these kinds of medications. One of the best is a combination of exercise and relaxation. Frederick Baekland, M.D., D.M.Sc., of the State University of New York, Brooklyn, reported that people who follow a regular exercise program experience more healthful, invigorating sleep than those who don't exercise.

Baekland used 14 student volunteers, recording their brain wave patterns during sleep for one month. During this time, the students, all physically active, were not permitted to exercise. Near the end of the month of exercise deprivation the students were asked to fill out questionnaires concerning their experiences and feelings during the test period.

In studying the electroencephalogram (EEG) charts and completed questionnaires, Baekland found that the most striking change was that the REM density (period of light sleep with much dreaming) increased remarkably in the students deprived of exercise. These students also reported more frequent awakenings during the night, a decrease in appetite, increases in sexual tension and the need to be with others. The EEG also recorded a higher number of body movements in the students. Perhaps this was their subconscious attempt to make up for the exercise they had lost.

Baekland's experiment also proved that the students who exercised daily were able to enjoy more deep sleep than the students who did not exercise. Students following their regular fitness program tended to awaken refreshed, and did not develop any of the psychological difficulties experienced by those students deprived of activity.

The study shows that if we don't exercise properly we're just too wound up to benefit from a night's sleep. We drag ourselves from bed every morning, our nerves jangled, our eyes baggy. We face each day with a growl instead of a smile. Yet by combining a program of intermittent relaxation with a sensible daily exercise routine, each of us would soon find ourself taking rapid steps to dreamland. An excellent approach is to modify the progressive relaxation technique described earlier in this chapter.

Most times insomnia occurs because of worry, tension, stress, and possibly other poor health habits. Here are some additional guidelines to help overcome insomnia.

1. Do not eat a heavy meal before going to bed.
2. Do not watch TV or read an exciting book before retiring.
3. Take a warm bath before retiring.
4. Drink a warm beverage just before bed.
5. Occupy yourself with a quiet hobby.
6. Take a leisurely walk before retiring.
7. Consciously try to relax the muscles of your body. Start with your feet and work your way up your body.
8. Get involved in a good overall aerobic fitness program.

The three Rs are basic to your energy needs. You can't go through life on hype. You need time to relax and recreate. You need time to recharge your batteries.

Your first Three Phase Plan follows. In this and the other plans, take the test to determine whether you should enter at Phase I, Phase II, or Phase III. Then, give the plans a chance. If you stay with a plan for two or three weeks, you will begin to notice positive changes in your energy levels.

A Three-Phase Plan for Enjoying Life

The following test will give you a fairly objective indication of how much you enjoy life. From the scoring on this test plus a general idea of how much you think you enjoy life, you can determine at what level you should begin to fight back.

Enjoyment of Life Test*

Directions: For each question, check Yes or No. If you feel that you do not know the answer, or if it is one half yes and one half no, check both yes and no.

		YES	NO
1.	Do people who know you well think you get upset easily?	❏	❏
2.	Do people who know you well think you are stubborn?	❏	❏
3.	Do people who know you well think you understand other people's points of view and accept them the way they are?	❏	❏
4.	Do people who know you well think that when you get mad you get over it quickly?	❏	❏
5.	Do people who know you well think you overcome problems easily?	❏	❏
6.	Do people who know you well think you are reliable and responsible in meeting your financial obligations?	❏	❏
7.	Do people who know you well think you have continued to mature and grow emotionally as you have gotten older?	❏	❏
8.	Do you like being among people, sharing interest in activity, going out socially?	❏	❏
9.	Do you think that changing your life in some way might make it easier to get well once you get sick?	❏	❏
10.	Is it reasonably easy for you to get to know people and make friends?	❏	❏
11.	Do you have good health?	❏	❏
12.	Do you think you had a satisfying religious education?	❏	❏
13.	Are you pleased when a friend is praised in your presence?	❏	❏
14.	Can you be friendly and sociable with the opposite sex without any feeling of awkwardness and strain?	❏	❏
15.	Do you think those close to you provide the emotional support you need?	❏	❏
16.	Can you take criticism and instruction in a good spirit?	❏	❏
17.	Are you satisfied with your occupation?	❏	❏
18.	Are you satisfied with your working conditions?	❏	❏
19.	Is your income satisfactory?	❏	❏
20.	Have you set goals for the future that satisfy you and are realistic?	❏	❏

Scoring: To score the test, give yourself +5 points for every Yes answer and -5 points for every No answer, except for questions 1 and 2. For these two questions, a No answer receives +5 points and a Yes answer receives -5 points. Where you've answered Yes and No to an item you receive 0 points. Determine your total score. It will lie somewhere between -100 and +100.

80 to 100	You seem to enjoy life—enter at Phase 3.
40 to 80	You're not sure you really enjoy life—enter at Phase 2.
Negative score to 40	You do not find life enjoyable—enter at Phase 1.

*SOURCE: Dr. Donald L. Dudley and Elton Welke, *How to Live with Stress*, Forum International Journal of Human Relations, November 1977, pp. 14-15.

Phase One: Identify the Sources of Stress in Your Life*

To help you more clearly understand some of the reasons why life may not be so enjoyable for you, check any of the following conditions that apply to you:

☐ 1. Too many people to relate to.
☐ 2. Frequent overtime and long hours.
☐ 3. Egotistical fellow employees or supervisors.
☐ 4. Excessive deadlines to meet.
☐ 5. Excessive technical and repetitive work.
☐ 6. Deluge of seemingly senseless paperwork.
☐ 7. Fear of the consequences of making mistakes.
☐ 8. Excessive noise.
☐ 9. Extreme smells, sights, heat, and cold.
☐ 10. Smoke and toxic substances in the air.
☐ 11. Feeling of incompetence.
☐ 12. Job seems meaningless and unchallenging.
☐ 13. Lack of true friends to share feelings with.
☐ 14. Current physical problems
☐ 15. Failing marriage.
☐ 16. Poor money management resulting in excessive debt.
☐ 17. Long drive to and from work and rush hour traffic.
☐ 18. Overcommitment to clubs, organizations, church, etc.
☐ 19. Strained relationships with the children.
☐ 20. Not enough time for recreation and hobbies.

ADDITIONAL CONDITIONS

☐ 21. _____
☐ 22. _____
☐ 23. _____
☐ 24. _____
☐ 25. _____

Now go over the list above and select the three major sources of stress in your life:

1. _____
2. _____
3. _____

---

*SOURCE: Adapted from Ron Clinton's stress inventory in *How to Prevent Burnout and Achieve Personal Well Being* Detroit: Human Potential Pub., 1980.

Phase Two: Attack One "Stress Target"

From the list of stress sources you selected in Phase One, select one as your "target" for one week. Plan an all-out attack on that target. Your plan will include the following components:

1. **DEVISE A REALISTIC TIME SCHEDULE.** There are many ways to do this. One simple method is to use 3" x 5" cards for each day of the week. On one side of the card, simply list your primary tasks and secondary tasks. On the other side, write down a time schedule for the day.

2. **APPROACH PRIMARY TASKS WITH A POSITIVE ATTITUDE.** As you write down your primary tasks, think or concentrate on the good that will happen when you finish the task. For example:

    PRIMARY TASK: Complete the refinishing job I started on the kitchen table and chairs.

    POSITIVE RESULTS: 1. Family won't have to eat on TV trays scattered throughout the house.

                           2. Will be able to put my kitchen back in order.

                           3. Will give me a sense of pride and accomplishment.

                           4. Will give me time to enjoy something else.

3. **TAKE TIME TO CONFIDE IN SOMEONE.** This, perhaps, will be the most difficult, but could also help you the most. Select someone you can trust and make it a point to spend some time with that individual for the sole purpose of sharing your feelings and emotions.

4. **TAKE CHARGE OF YOUR PROBLEMS.** Write down one major problem you must face this week:

    _____

    Now list at least three ways of handling that problem. Do not include "ignoring it" as an option.

    _____

    _____

    _____

    Select what you think is the best option and apply that solution to the problem.

5. **ANTICIPATE OBSTACLES THAT MAY STOP YOU.** Beat those obstacles to the punch. If you think about them ahead of time, you will already have an idea of how to get around them. Write down any obstacles that you think will stand in your way:

    _____

    _____

    _____

6. **MEET THOSE OBSTACLES HEAD-ON.** For any of the obstacles that you selected, write down how you plan to get around those obstacles.

    _____

    _____

    _____

7. **RECOGNIZE YOUR OWN PERSONAL VALUE.** Begin or end each day by thinking about those things about you that make you proud of yourself. This can be done while commuting to work, jogging or walking, or lying in bed.

Phase Three: Make the Fight Enjoyable

In the first phase you got a handle on the cause of your stress. In Phase Two you began to fight back. In Phase Three you will continue the fight by adding other "stress targets" to your hit list. But now, you are beginning to master your problems. The fight is now becoming a challenge. Instead of looking at life as a series of problems to overcome, you view each day as a challenge and find excitement in trying to meet that challenge. Some things that will help you turn the fight into a challenge are included below:

REST If you ignore this element, you may not have enough energy to keep up with your enjoyable lifestyle.

1. Go to bed one half-hour earlier than normal. If you aren't tired enough to sleep, use the time to read, write letters, talk with your spouse, or listen to music.

2. If you are using a sleeping aid such as a barbiturate or a tranquilizer, stop for at least a two-week trial period. If you have difficulty sleeping during that time, try some of these methods.

   A. Drink a cup of warm milk or herb tea one half-hour before retiring.

   B. Read something that is not related in any way to your work. Fiction is usually better for this than nonfiction.

   C. Exercise leisurely for 10 minutes just before going to bed.

   D. Take a hot bath before you retire.

   E. Practice a relaxation technique while lying in bed.

   F. Try falling asleep to soft music.

   G. Sip a half glass of wine 20 minutes before retiring. (Caution: if you are a regular moderate to heavy drinker, this will be of no help. Most alcoholics are plagued with insomnia.)

   H. Do not drink any coffee, tea, cola, or eat chocolate after noon.

RECREATION Put the play back into your life...even if it means being a kid again.

1. If you do not already do it, perform an aerobic activity (jogging, walking, swimming, etc.) for at least 20 minutes a day three times a week.

2. Once each week, participate in a noncompetitive physical activity with your family or friends. Suggested activities include:

Free-form wrestling and tumbling	Skiing (snow or water)
Imitate animal motions	Canoeing or sailing
Backyard obstacle course	Archery
Playground equipment play	Tree climbing
Dancing	Horseback riding
Hiking (on foot or bike)	Skating (ice or roller)
Sledding and tobogganing	Ping-Pong and badminton

NOTE: Traditional recreational activities like golf, bowling, softball, etc., are fine if a) competition does not become serious, b) a regular obligation does not turn it into a chore, c) relationships with family and/or friends do not play second fiddle to the activity.

RELAXATION Practice daily at least one of the relaxation techniques outlined in Chapter 8.

▶▶*Enjoying Fitness* ▶ ▶ ▶ ▶

LSD and the O₂ High ▶▶ ▶▶

I've been coming down hard on drugs all through this book, so you're probably surprised that now I'm recommending LSD. But I do recommend it. To me, LSD refers to Long Slow Distance. That's the best way to acquire the O_2 High.

This is not a lot of hocus-pocus I'm giving you. I really believe in getting high on O_2—oxygen. And the best way to get this type of "high" is through aerobic activities.

Aerobic Activity

Over twenty years ago, Dr. Kenneth Cooper, author of *Aerobics,* began using the word that has since become a household term for people who exercise. That word is "aerobic," meaning "with oxygen." I have found that participating in vigorous activities that use large amounts of oxygen (activities that make you huff and puff) will help you develop a boundless supply of energy. To me, aerobic exercise is the foundation of any energy plan.

Let's take a close look at aerobic exercise. Just what do I mean when I toss that concept around? In my travels throughout the United States and Canada, I've observed a rapid increase in the activity levels of most people. Practically everyone owned a double-knit jogging suit when they were in style. Tennis courts are being built at a rapid rate, yet it's still difficult to find an empty court. Athletic facilities are in use almost 24 hours a day. Ditto for racquetball, handball, and squash courts. Ten years ago, you could mention the word Reebok and few would know you were referring to an athletic shoe company. Now, at cocktail parties and church socials it is not uncommon to hear lively debate on the merits of Nike over L.A. Gear. It seems as if everyone is climbing aboard the fitness wagon.

And that's good! It's good, except for one thing. Most of the activities that people choose are not aerobic. They are good, wholesome, fun activities, but they do little to increase your innate supply of energy. If you are concerned with getting more energy out of each minute, you need to spend some time each or every other day with one of the big four: running, walking, swimming, or cycling. Other energy-building activities are cross-country skiing and ice or roller skating. These are activities which can be done slowly, for a long period of time.

As you can see, these activities all have something in common. They are rhythmic and sustained. They are not too strenuous, which means you can keep at them for 20 minutes to an hour. You never reach a point of total exhaustion, though your pulse increases, your breathing is heavier, and you may sweat a bit. That's what aerobic exercise is all about. Any activity that demands a steady use of oxygen for at least 20 minutes is considered aerobic.

In contrast, most sports and leisure-time activities do not meet those requirements. They are either too hard or too easy. Take, for example, tennis. I really enjoy a game of tennis, even though I'm not very good. But I seldom get a real workout from a tennis game. Even if I play several games over an hour or so, I seldom have to breathe hard for more than five minutes at a time. Consequently, my activity is not aerobic.

Another popular activity is weight lifting, yet this activity does not qualify as aerobic because it's too hard. Most lifting is done in sets. That is, the lifter will pump the iron seven to ten times, then rest. You have to rest or you'd simply drop. That's because weight lifting places a heavy demand on selected muscles, not your whole body. It is impossible to steadily lift weights for 20 to 30 minutes. Your muscles would not permit you to do it.

Don't get me wrong. These are fine activities and it's encouraging to see more and more people choosing an active way of life over a more sedentary lifestyle. I love to play handball and tennis and I lift weights regularly. These activities build some energy. For example, the tennis and handball allow me to get the competitive urges out of me. They also help me release some anger. Whacking a ball hard helps me release a lot of tension and frustration in a socially acceptable way.

My weight-training conditions different muscles. Well-toned muscles make my body look better. If my body looks better, that gives me a psychological lift. I feel good about the way I look. Also, that lift, believe it or not, gives me energy.

Additionally, vigorous exercise of any type will cause a temporary lift because of possible biochemical changes. But more on that later in this chapter.

I want to emphasize that a nonaerobic activity may not give you energy in the same way as an aerobic activity. It may even contribute to the energy drain that's been bothering you, simply because you're not in shape to play the sport. If the tennis match leaves you feeling sore, worn out, and tired the next day, it's because you're simply not in adequate condition to play it.

What special qualities of aerobic exercise make it the energy builder it is? There are many, including an increase in oxygen uptake, reduction in body fat, stress transfer, anger and anxiety abatement, a lift out of depression, and increased productivity and creativity.

Oxygen Uptake

I told you earlier that aerobics meant "with oxygen.".As you know, human life depends upon oxygen. Without it we die. Similarly, with reduced amounts of it we are slowed down. When the human body becomes inefficient in transporting oxygen to various parts of the body, a lack of energy occurs.

Oxygen permits your muscles to contract, your brain to think, and your digestive system to digest. Of course, most people are able to take in enough oxygen to "get through" the day. But unless you have good aerobic capacity, your efficiency in handling oxygen is not what it should be.

Proper amounts of oxygen permit your cells and tissues to work in an efficient manner. Oxygen is delivered to your tissues by means of your heart, blood, and blood vessels. When you are fit, your circulatory system becomes more efficient. Regular aerobic exercise may:

1. Increase the number and size of your blood vessels for better and more efficient circulation.

2. Increase the elasticity of the blood vessels, thereby permitting more blood to be circulated.

3. Increase the efficiency of exercising muscles and blood circulation so that muscles and blood are better able to pick up, carry, and use oxygen.

4. Increase the efficiency of the heart, making it able to pump more blood with fewer beats.

5. Increase the number of red blood cells so that more oxygen can be carried throughout your body.

These five benefits, plus some other complicated biochemical changes over a period of weeks and months, permit your body to improve its ability to pick up, deliver, and use oxygen. The result is more oxygen available to the tissues. And more oxygen to the tissues means more energy. It's as though you have been transformed from being a gas guzzler of the 60's and early 70's to being a fuel-efficient automobile of the 90's. You get more mileage from the same amount of energy.

A report by Dr. Roy J. Shephard, of the University of Toronto, Department of Physiological Hygiene, notes that an individual's aerobic fitness capacity typically declines with age. By 60, many men and most women are unable to work an eight-hour day without suffering from fatigue. But, says Dr. Shephard, "through the use of an appropriate training program (aerobic exercise), it is possible to improve working capacity by at least 15 or 20 percent." Working capacity, of course, has to do with endurance and stamina. You are able to do more before feeling fatigue. True energy begins with aerobic fitness.

Reduction of Body Fat

One of the most obvious reasons for lack of energy is obesity. Many Americans work too hard because they carry around excess body fat. From the ages of 20 to 50, the average American gains between 1 to 2 pounds of fat a year. This extra fat robs you of energy.

A bag of groceries weighs about 15 pounds. That's really not too heavy, but if for some reason you had to carry that bag any further than from the market to the car, you would get fatigued.

Most people are no more than 10 to 15 pounds overfat, and yet that additional weight is enough to leave them feeling tired and run down. Instead of being able to "set the package down" and take a little rest, the overfat are forced to carry the weight all of their waking hours. No wonder they run out of energy so quickly—and avoid activity.

It doesn't have to be that way. If aerobic exercise did nothing else, the benefits from fat loss would be enough to give you noticeable extra energy to help you enjoy more of each minute, and give you an extra hour or two of "fun time" after you get home from work. This energy can make your day at the office or plant more productive, and it comes from not having to carry around extra fat.

Aerobic exercise is the best way to reduce energy-wasting fat. To lose fat, you simply make sure you use more calories than you eat. That's simple enough. And, you have two ways to do this: diet or exercise. Dieting works, sometimes. But eventually the fat comes back because the regimen of a strict diet is too difficult for most humans. That's because we must eat to live. Therefore, most diets rob you of energy. Additionally, researchers say that when you diet to lose weight you lose bone, muscle, and organ tissue as well as fat. And while those lost pounds may look good on the scale, they rob you of vital energy. Muscles give you go power! Your organs (brain included) need the proper number of cells to give you optimum energy. But fat robs you of it all.

A more sensible way to drop that unwanted load of fat without losing bone, muscle, and organ tissue is to burn off those extra calories through aerobic exercise. Exercise that's aerobic in nature removes the fat more quickly and more consistently. Why? By spending a half-hour a day, four to five days per week in an activity like bicycling, you will lose from 1,400 to 1,750 calories per week. Since 3,500 calories roughly equal one pound, in ten days you'll have dropped a pound. In just under three weeks, two pounds. Keep it up for six months and you will have dropped ten pounds. And that's with absolutely no change in your eating habits!

Exercise has been shown to have a positive effect on your emotional and mental health as well. By proven ways (and ways yet to be discovered), exercise increases your energy level substantially. These include transfer of stress and anger; abatement of anxiety; lifting of depression; and improvement of creativity and confidence.

Stress Transfer

I'm sure you've heard people say: "This job gives me a headache," or "I'm so mad my blood is boiling." These statements are quite correct. Frustrations, anger, hostilities, and headaches can create high blood pressure and other energy-robbing diseases—but a change in activity can help a person master those feelings. I want to show you here how exercise, specifically aerobic exercise, can give you mental and emotional energy.

A study conducted by Drs. John Boyer, M.D., and Fred Kasch, Ph.D., on 23 middle-aged men with high blood pressure and 23 men with normal blood pressure demonstrated the effectiveness of six months of exercise on blood pressure. (High blood pressure robs people of personal energy.) The test subjects' routine consisted of 15 to 20 minutes of warm-up exercises, followed by walking and jogging. All of these men had been inactive before the program, and no attempt was made to alter their diet. At the end of the six months, there were significant reductions in the blood pressure of the hypertensive men.

Energy-robbing neuromuscular headaches can also be relieved through physical activity. A study conducted by Dr. Herbert deVries of the

Gerontology Center at the University of California illustrates this nicely. Working with a group of men 50 years and older, all of whom had a history of migraine headaches, deVries found that after a few weeks of regular physical activity, the headaches disappeared—without medication.

Anger and Anxiety Abatement

Exercise can also play an important role in helping to relieve anger and anxiety. Earlier I shared with you that swatting a handball is good therapy for me. It relieves my frustrations. I know hundreds of other YMCA personnel who have told me the same thing. A vigorous game of racquetball, basketball, or volleyball helps them temper their hostilities and frustrations in a socially acceptable way.

Dr. William P. Morgan, researcher on emotions and exercise at the University of Wisconsin, noted that after a vigorous workout there is a measurable decrease in anxiety. The level of adrenaline in the blood, the blood pressure, and the heart rate are also reduced. Clinically, many people report improved feelings and less anxiety after a good bout of strenuous exercise.

While it is difficult at the present time to determine how exercise improves the mind and why it reduces anger and anxiety, it probably will be demonstrated in the future that the brain's nerve transmitters are changed in some way that causes people to feel better and more vigorous.

In addition to walking, running, or swatting handballs, there are other ways in which negative emotions caused by stress can be transformed into useful energy. Therapist Laura Archera Huxley claims this can be done through any kind of consciously directed muscular activity. She advocates kicking or squeezing a tether ball, or at moments when one experiences stress but cannot react openly to it, repeatedly contracting muscle groups that one wishes to strengthen or beautify for ten seconds, then relaxing them. For example, the abdomen, thighs, or derriere. Such isometric exercises will convert anger or anxiety that's otherwise destined to cause physical or emotional problems into greater fitness and well-being. We thus can become "expert voluntary energy transformers instead of involuntary energy victims."

I think Dr. Allan Clark of St. Joseph's Infirmary in Atlanta, Ga., summarizes it best: "It is well known that exercise is the best tranquilizer. I refuse to medicate patients with simple neurotic anxiety until they have given aerobic exercise an adequate trial."

Depression and Blues

As mentioned earlier, psychologists and psychiatrists are now looking at exercise, specifically running, as an option to help people handle the blues, or mild depression. For some reason, running seems to be a mood elevator. Studies at the University of Virginia among students who claimed to suffer from depression showed that those who worked out vigorously three times a week for ten weeks had an improvement in their scores on tests designed to measure depression. Working out lifted their feelings. The wrestlers, the joggers, the exercisers, and tennis players all noted this mood elevation. But those who played softball did not. It is entirely possible that softball simply isn't vigorous enough to reduce depression.

Another study done at the University of Wisconsin under the direction of Dr. John Griest compared running with psychotherapy. In this study people who came to the clinic were assigned to ten weeks of running therapy, ten weeks of psychotherapy, or to unlimited psychotherapy. The running group had to hoof it with their therapist three times a week. Talk of depression was discouraged during the run. If the patient persisted in discussing it, the leader suggested the patient focus on running and breathing instead. At the end of the experiment, the running patients and those in the ten-week psychotherapy group showed the most improvement. Significantly, a year later most of the joggers were still running and were free of depression.

"I have often started out a walk in a state called mad," said Donald Culors Pattie. "Mad in the sense of soreheaded, or mad with tedium or confusion; I have set forth dull, null, and even thoroughly discouraged but I never came back in such a frame of mind, and I have never met a human being that was not better for a walk." This is equally true of other forms of exercise.

Creativity

One of the reasons I exercise is because my head calls for it. I may be happy to get the benefits derived from looking better and feeling healthier, but as far as I'm concerned they are only side effects. The real reason is mental or emotional. Exercise adds life to my years. It improves my creativity.

About 30 minutes into a run, my creative juices really start to flow. The LSD starts to take effect. I solve all kinds of administrative, writing, family, and personal problems in a short period of time. Most of my book, program, and article ideas have come on the run. I agree with Dr. George Sheehan who has said, "Never trust an idea that you have sitting down." When my run is finished I am tired physically. But I am full of creative energy.

Dr. Thaddeus Kostrubala, the running psychiatrist mentioned earlier, notes that as a runner approaches the 30-minute mark, he feels depressed.

Some subjects even told him that at the 30-minute mark they feel like crying and occasionally do. Perhaps it is pain, perhaps it is the desire for sympathy. But a short time after the 30-minute mark is reached, some people experience an "opening-up phenomenon." Their breathing becomes easier, their legs feel stronger, and they feel almost euphoric.

Now Kostrubala admits this is a pretty amazing phenomenon. His explanation deals with the left and right sides of the brain. The left side controls the functional aspects of day-to-day living, while the right side controls, among other things, creative functions. The only problem is that to break through to that right side takes some doing. In a sense, we have to escape one level of consciousness to give the brain a clear slate from which to produce new ideas—to create. This level of consciousness is often approached through various forms of repetition.

Kostrubala maintains that the repetitive nature of running, along with whatever repetition you intone mentally with each step, helps you to reach this level of consciousness. He suggests that after 30 or 40 minutes of slow, long-distance, repetitive running, the left side of the brain gets bored and lets the right side of the brain take over. In other words, you have more creative energy. Of course, that phenomenon need not be confined to running. Walking, swimming, bicycling, and cross-country skiing will elicit the same response.

A lot of times our busy schedules prevent us from periods of reflection necessary to the creative process. The calm solitude of exercising alone gives you a chance to work things out in your mind. New ideas to help you approach an old problem are more likely to pop into your head while you are running, cycling, or walking, than if you were spending the same time watching TV or worrying about that problem.

Confidence

Good fitness builds confidence as well. Dr. Thomas K. Cureton, the grandaddy of fitness in the U.S.A., says this is one of the greatest benefits of exercise. His exhaustive work at the University of Illinois over four decades convinced him that most middle-aged men lose confidence in their physical ability as they get older. They become unfit, have sagging waistlines, flabby muscles, gain weight, and are breathless under exertion. Since men are taught early in life that manliness and physical vigor go hand in hand, their self-confidence slips, and their mental and emotional well-being are affected as well.

Cureton maintains that through exercise men will lose their timidity. As their narrow waistline returns, weight drops, muscles firm up, and stamina improves, they become physical beings once more. Exercise helps them to reestablish their self-confidence.

How to Do It

I hope by now you are excited enough about gaining more energy through aerobic exercise to give it a try. But don't just lace on a pair of sneakers and head for the hills. Unfortunately, too many people get all hyped up about exercise, overdo it, then suffer minor problems like blisters and aching muscles. Then they give up. Therefore, you need to approach your exercise program more realistically. To begin, establish how much, how hard, and how often you should exercise.

How Much

Don't get hung up on distance. Many people, when they begin a walking or jogging program, measure their distance, but miles don't mean a thing to your body. Minutes do. If you have been inactive for at least a year, I suggest setting a goal of 20 to 30 minutes of aerobic activity. If it's longer than that, you will probably push too hard and suffer some minor aches and pains. As you become more proficient and your fitness level increases, you can increase that time up to an hour a day if you choose. However, as far as increased energy and general fitness is concerned, 30 to 40 minutes of aerobic exercise each session is an adequate amount, with at least 20 minutes at your target heart rate.

How Hard

You have an amazing mechanism for determining how hard to exercise: your pulse. Therefore learn to listen to your body, starting with your wrist. Use the second, third, and fourth fingers of one hand to feel for the pulse along the thumb-side of your other wrist. Take your pulse rate for ten seconds. Then multiply that count by six to find how many times your heart beats per minute.

Take your pulse now. You'll probably find it's between 60 and 80 beats per minute. It's relatively easy to take your pulse while sitting, but when exercising, you'll have to slow down for a few seconds, check your pulse, and then resume your activity.

How does this tell you how hard you should exercise? Your ideal exercise level is determined by your target heart rate. Your target heart rate is approximately 60 to 85 percent of your maximum heart rate (see chart on the next page). To make sure you are exercising hard enough, check your pulse occasionally to see if your heart rate falls within the target zone. The maximum heart rate of a young child is around 200 beats per minute, and since physiologists tell us that our maximum heart rate drops about one beat a year, you can subtract your age from the maximum number of 220 beats per minute. So if you are 40 years of age, figure 60 to 85 percent of that number. This is how the target heart rate chart below was determined.

AGE	TARGET HEART RATE (BEATS PER MINUTE)
10-19	125 to 180
20-29	120 to 170
30-39	115 to 160
40-49	110 to 150
50-59	100 to 145
60-69	95 to 135

You also can determine whether you are exercising too hard by listening to other parts of your body. If your breathing is extremely labored, or if you feel a tightness or pain in your chest or shoulder, then slow down. Note whether you are able to hold a conversation while exercising. If you are breathing so hard that you can't talk, then you are working too hard.

By listening to your body you can forget trying to beat the clock, one of the most destructive forces in a personal energy exercise program. If you figure two miles in 17 minutes is good, then two miles in 15 minutes must be better; that kind of thinking will drain your energy, not build it. Think in terms of exercising for a period of time when you feel good. Constantly pushing yourself to be number one can drain you physically and frustrate you.

Remember, you are exercising for maximum personal energy, not for sport. Your goal in building energy is to go long and slow.

How Often

You simply must commit yourself to a three days per week minimum if you desire to increase your energy level. While some people try to exercise every day of the week, usually a day or two of rest is advisable, especially if you have been inactive for some time. Thus, your prescription for higher energy through aerobic exercise should include 20 to 40 minutes of target heart rate exercise three to six days a week.

Stretch for Energy ▶**10**▶▶

If you were not allowed to stretch at all for a week, you'd begin to feel like a walking time bomb. Tension would mount, muscles would become impossibly stiff, and your range of motion would be severely restricted. You would bc seriously affected emotionally and psychologically, as well as physically. The stretch reflex allows you to relax.

Human beings love to stretch; we can't cope with life for long without stretching, and fortunately, stretching is very good for us. A little stretching is essential, and a lot of stretching, if done properly, can result in greater physical efficiency, coordination, agility, balance, and quickness; a vastly improved range of motion; and most importantly, a release of muscle tension. It is the best insurance you can have against injury. Proper stretching is one of the best relaxation techniques there is.

Athletes are dedicated stretchers, primarily because they know it's the best way to avoid winding up being carried off the field on a stretcher. Most torn ligaments, pulled muscles, and other bodily injuries due to vigorous movement could be prevented by a proper warm-up that includes careful stretching of the various muscle groups.

So stretch for energy, because there's nothing like an injury (or disease) to make you suddenly feel energy-deficient. If just a hangnail can make you feel bad all over, imagine what Achilles tendonitis will do for your energy level.

I recommend ten minutes of stretching as part of the warm-up before any aerobic activity, to reduce the possibility of injury. Following the workout, stretch for ten minutes as part of your cool-down to prevent stiff, sore muscles, and to help you relax. In fact, though the injury prevention qualities of proper stretching cannot be overemphasized, it's the contribution stretching makes to relaxation that most fascinates me. You can stretch to relax, and the result will be less tension, less fatigue, less exhaustion. In fact, many people who practice stretching, yoga, or similar kinds of activities report that afterwards they are more vigorous and alert. In other words, they have more energy.

The Benefits of Stretching

The main job of your muscles is to tighten or contract. Contractions allow limbs to move so you can run, walk, sit, stand, eat, write, type, and drive. Tension is normal and necessary for every move you make. Of course, muscles are not to be tense or contracted all the time. When sitting, the muscles of your upper legs are generally relaxed, as are your abdominal muscles. But your lower back and lower leg muscles are contracted to help you sit properly. When lying down, however, your thigh muscles are contracted and your back muscles are relaxed. This beautiful interplay of muscles relaxing, contracting, and partially contracting or relaxing allows you to function efficiently and smoothly with minimum fatigue.

The muscles are usually the first sign of tension. Before you have a headache, stomach pain, or whipped feeling, your muscles warn you with an eye twitch, a neck or back pain, or muscle fatigue.

Problems result when muscles tense up and there is no need for the tension. There's no reason for your back muscles to be tight when you're lying down. However, many people remain tense even in prone positions, which explains why low back pain is one of the major complaints doctors hear these days. A majority of back problems are the result of weak or inflexible muscles, muscles that stay tight even though they ought to be relaxing.

To find out if your muscles are too tense, pay attention to these warning signs:

1. Do you have eye twitches?
2. Do you have neck or low back pain?
3. Do you have restless legs (you feel as though you must get up and walk about frequently)?
4. Do you seem to clench your fists repeatedly? Or do you hold the phone or steering wheel of your car very tightly?
5. Do your muscles seem to tire easily when performing a physical task—such as typing and writing?

6. Do you seem to lack flexibility at different joints of your body? When you try to touch your toes do your back and leg muscles rebel?

7. Upon awakening, does it seem as though your jaw is tired as a result of gritting or clenching your teeth?

8. Do you find that you have been very rigid in your sleeping?

9. Does your spouse tell you that you twitch or jump a great deal?

All of these are symptoms of muscle tension. And if they occur infrequently, it's not too much of a problem. But if they appear often during a week, then you know that you're probably experiencing too much muscle tension.

Once you've discovered that you have muscle tension and fatigue, it's time to use stretching for relaxation, reducing fatigue, and hence, building energy.

The Two Types of Stretching

Exercise physiologists tell us there are two basic stretching methods: ballistic and static. Ballistic stretching involves bouncing and bobbing to see how close you can come to touching your toes. Static stretching is the slow, easy approach where you gradually reach down to the point where you feel a tug on your muscles. At that point you hold. Then you concentrate on the tight muscle groups, trying to get these muscles to relax. The muscles usually relax and then you can slip down a little bit further to another point of tug or slight discomfort, then hold. The result is an improvement of flexibility, the by-product of relaxed muscles.

Opinions differ on which is best—ballistic or static stretching. Ballistic stretching is the old "hup...two...three...four" routine. Recently, static stretching has been employed with good success among professional athletic teams. In fact, it has become so pervasive among athletic teams that many have rejected the old ballistic routines.

To discover which approach is best, Dr. Herbert deVries of the University of Southern California undertook an investigation. His research concluded that static stretching is just as effective as the old-fashioned ballistic method, but with three distinct advantages:

1. Static stretching poses less danger of exceeding the extensibility limits of the tissues involved (less chance of injury and pain).

2. Static stretching requires less energy.

3. Static stretching generally relieves sore muscles, rather than causing them.

Interestingly, deVries also discovered that the improvements brought about by static stretching persisted for a longer period of time—eight weeks and more—after the stretching program was discontinued. Significantly, stretching can improve the flexibility and relaxation ability in the old as well as in the young.

If you are familiar with exercise, you'll probably recognize that static stretching is similar to the classic yoga poses, postures, and concepts. And it is the static stretch that I recommend for a warm-up prior to aerobic exercise and cool-down after exercise. I also recommend static stretching as a relaxation technique.

Back in the 1960's, in their quest for a more fulfilled life, reduced tension, and a desire for greater energy reserves, many Americans turned to yoga. There are many varieties of yoga, but the most popular type is Hatha Yoga. In Hatha (physical) Yoga, a series of postures (asanas) consisting of stretching, balancing, standing, and sitting postures is employed. A yoga workout typically combines groups of these postures (to stretch most major muscle groups), the movements of getting into and out of them, relaxation, and simple breathing exercises. A great deal of emphasis is placed on static stretching.

The benefits derived from regular static stretching or a program of Hatha Yoga are similar. Remember, however, that yogis spend long hours in static stretch positions in their quest to obtain these benefits. I feel similar benefits may be derived by holding the static stretch position for no more than a minute or so. Devote the time you save to an activity that burns calories and has a training effect on your heart and lungs. Ultimately this will build greater energy.

To derive the most benefit from stretching, be sure to do it correctly. First, prior to the stretch, walk for five minutes or so. As you walk, move your arms in giant circles, forward and backward. These movements will help increase your body temperature, so that your body is properly prepared for stretching. Do each stretch slowly and without straining. Don't worry if you cannot achieve the extreme positions of the super-flexible individual. Stretch only as far as is comfortable. While you are holding that position, relax. When you feel tension in a particular muscle, concentrate on relaxing it. Remarkably, this advice on stretching in yoga is parallel to the results suggested by deVries's research: the stretch is to be slow, sustained, and not ballistic.

Research, logic, and experience indicate that yoga exercises are very effective in improving flexibility. Caution must be exercised, however, not to get into extreme positions without proper conditioning. The same is true of other stretches. Extreme postures are not necessary for the average person.

However, don't avoid stretching entirely. Anyone on an aerobic program of running, walking, or cycling should use selected static stretch exercises for flexibility development.

Paul Uram, the flex coach for the Pittsburgh Steelers, has made many suggestions and observations about proper stretching, some of which follow.

1. Do not force your muscles to stretch more than they are ready for, and don't progress too rapidly.

2. When stretching one set of muscles, also stretch the opposite set. That is, when you stretch the hamstring muscles on the back of your legs, also stretch the quadricep muscles on the front.

3. The functioning of one muscle group is almost always related to the functioning of another group, so stretches to help the back may also benefit both leg and shoulder muscles.

4. Keep warm while stretching. This enhances all of the benefits of static stretches.

5. Learn to recognize the tension, discomfort, and occasional pain that accompany stretching, and use them to your advantage. This feedback can help you recognize how far you can safely stretch. While performing a given stretch, go just far enough to feel the stretch but not so far that you feel pain.

6. Relax while stretching. Don't hold your breath. Breathe normally. Rather than fighting the exercise, relax your way through it.

7. Hold stretches for short periods of time at first and then progress to longer holds.

8. DO NOT BOUNCE. Bouncing does not allow the muscle time to benefit from the stretch, and may cause injury. Also, bouncing actually causes the muscle to contract rather than to adapt to the stretched length, due to what is called the stretch reflex.

9. If you do not have the flexibility and poise of a gymnast, don't let that stop you from beginning a stretch program. Just stretch your muscles, and learn to like that stretching feeling.

As far as I'm concerned, aerobic exercise and static stretching make the perfect marriage for building energy. One builds energy by increasing the oxygen-carrying capacity of your body, building better muscle tone, developing a better cardiovascular system that functions more efficiently, reducing your body fat, helping reduce the blues, and giving an outlet for removing your anger and anxiety. Static stretching, on the other hand, complements aerobic exercise and gives you an opportunity to maintain your flexibility so that you can do plenty of aerobic exercise for true relaxation. Plus, it winds you down from the hype of a busy life.

Many aerobic exercisers forget the importance of stretching. They go into the activity full bore. In my fitness classes I see many people who rush in from work, get into their gym shorts, and bound up to the gymnasium to start doing their laps. As soon as the aerobic exercise is finished, they rush back to the locker room, down a few glasses of juice or a cup of yogurt, and dash off again. While they may be building aerobic fitness, they have done nothing to help prevent injury. On top of it they have not really relaxed. While they're building one type of aerobic energy, I'm afraid they're just adding more hype to their life. Stretching provides that opportunity.

Yogis are many times at fault as well. They forget about aerobic exercise. They think stretching will do it all. Stretching will provide relaxation. But they forget that a more healthful cardiovascular system will help to build energy by increasing their body's ability to pick up and transport oxygen.

So put the two together. Stretch and become fit aerobically.

Stretching Techniques

Below are a series of stretches that I recommend. These stretches are followed by a three-phase program for improving energy via exercise.

Moderate Stretching Exercises

SINGLE LEG TUCK—Sit on the floor with your left leg straight and your right leg bent. Tuck your right foot into your groin. Bend from the waist, reach forward, and clasp your left ankle. Pull your chest toward your left knee. Hold. Repeat with the right leg.

CALF TENDON STRETCHER—Stand 2 to 3 feet from the wall. Lean forward, body straight. Place palms against the wall at eye level. Step backward. Continue to support your weight with hands. Remain flat-footed until you feel calf muscles stretching.

STANDING LEG STRETCHER—Find a chair or table 2 feet in height. Place left foot on the chair or table. Keep this leg slightly bent and parallel to the floor. Your right leg should be planted firmly on the floor. From this position, slowly extend your fingertips toward your outstretched leg on the chair. Hold and return. Repeat with your other leg.

SIDE-TO-SIDE STRETCH—Stand with feet shoulder-width apart, left hand at your side, right hand extended over your head. Slowly bend at the waist toward your left. Reach down your leg with your left hand. Try to get your upper body parallel to the floor. Hold for eight to ten seconds, then repeat in the other direction.

CAT STRETCH—Get on your hands and knees and take a few relaxing breaths. Then, curl your chin to your chest while arching your back. Hold that position for eight to ten seconds, then relax.

ELBOW SPECIAL—Stand with your hands behind your head, fingers interlocked. Draw your elbows back as far as possible and hold. Draw the elbows forward and try to touch them together. Hold and repeat.

SHOULDER STRETCH—With your arms over your head, hold the elbow of one arm with the hand of the other arm. Slowly pull the elbow behind your head. Do not force. Hold. Repeat on the other side.

KNEELING SHOULDER STRETCH—Kneel on the floor, sit back on your heels, and look at your knees as you reach forward with your hands. Keep your seat down and continue to focus on your knees. Once you have reached as far as possible, press down against the floor with your hands. You will feel your shoulders stretch. Hold and repeat.

BEND AND STRETCH—While standing, clasp hands behind your waist. As you slowly bend forward at the waist, lift your arms, keeping the elbows slightly bent. When you begin to feel slight pressure, stop and hold. Return to starting position.

KNEE TO CHEST—Lie on the floor with your knees bent. Draw one knee to the chest by pulling on the back of the thigh with the hands. Then extend the leg toward the ceiling. Hold. Pull the knee to the chest again and return to the starting position. Repeat with the other leg.

A Three-Phase Plan for Enjoying Fitness

Take the following tests to see how fit you are.

COOPER'S THREE-MILE WALKING TEST (TIME IS DISPLAYED IN MINUTES)

FITNESS CATEGORY		AGE (YEARS)					
		13-19	20-29	30-39	40-49	50-59	60+
I. Very Poor							
	(Men)	>45:00*	>46:00	>49:00	>52:00	>55:00	>60:00
	(Women)	>47:00	>48:00	>51:00	>54:00	>57:00	>63:00
II. Poor							
	(Men)	41:01-45:00	42:01-46:00	44:31-49:00	47:01-52:00	50:01-55:00	54:01-60:00
	(Women)	43:01-47:00	44:01-48:00	46:31-51:00	49:01-54:00	52:01-57:00	57:01-63:00
III. Fair							
	(Men)	37:31-41:00	38:31-42:00	40:01-44:30	42:01-47:00	45:01-50:00	48:01-54:00
	(Women)	39:31-43:00	40:31-44:00	42:01-46:30	44:01-49:00	47:01-52:00	51:01-57:00
IV. Good							
	(Men)	33:00-37:30	34:00-38:30	35:00-40:00	36:30-42:00	39:00-45:00	41:00-48:00
	(Women)	35:00-39:30	36:00-40:30	37:30-42:00	39:00-44:00	42:00-47:00	45:00-51:00
V. Excellent							
	(Men)	<33:00	<34:00	<35:00	<36:30	<39:00	<41:00
	(Women)	<35:00	<36:00	<37:30	<39:00	<42:00	<45:00

SOURCE: Kenneth H. Cooper, *The Aerobics Way*, New York: M. Evans and Co.

NOTE: *The Walking Test,* covering three miles in the fastest time possible *without running,* can be done on a track over any accurately measured distance. As with running, take the test after you have been training for at least six weeks, when you feel rested, and when you are dressed comfortably.

*< means "less than"; > means "more than."

STANDARD FLEXIBILITY TEST (SIT AND REACH TEST)

MATERIALS:	yardstick and adhesive tape.
PROCEDURE:	1. Warm up with some stretching before the test.
	2. Sit on the floor with the legs extended and the heels about 5 inches apart.
	3. With a strip of masking tape, mark where the heels touch the floor.
	4. Place the yardstick on the floor between and parallel to the legs so that the 15-inch mark touches the near edge of the taped heel line.
	5. Slowly reach with both hands as far forward as possible. Touch the fingertips to the yardstick and hold this position momentarily. The yardstick shows the distance reached. Do not attempt to add length by jerking forward.
	6. Try the test three times, recording the distance in inches each time: _____, _____, _____ . Circle your best score.
	7. Check your scores with the norms provided on the next page.

Rating	Men (Inches)	Women (Inches)
Excellent	22-23	24-27
Good	20-21	21-23
Average	14-18	16-20
Fair	12-13	13-15
Poor	0-11	0-12

SOURCE: C.R. Myers, *The Official YMCA Physical Fitness Handbook*, New York: Popular Library, 1975, pp. 103-104.

The point on the plan at which you begin depends upon your score in the Three-Mile Walking Test. If you scored Very Poor or Poor, begin at Phase One. If you scored Fair or Good, begin at Phase Two. If you scored Excellent, begin at Phase Three unless it seems too taxing. In that event, begin about halfway through Phase Two.

Phase One

FLEXIBILITY   Spend five minutes a day doing five of the stretching exercises described in Chapter 10.

AEROBIC FITNESS   Spend at least one week on each of the following levels, trying to do the activity at least three times each week. If you move up to the next level after a week and it seems too difficult, drop back to the previous level for another week. When you walk, walk at a comfortable yet steady pace. Because you are not in peak physical condition, the most important lesson you can learn is patience. Moving too rapidly through the levels may result in discomfort or injury.

NUMBER OF MINUTES TO WALK PER DAY

10-20
20-25
25-30
30-35
35-40
40-45

Spend a *minimum* of one week at each of these levels.

Phase Two

FLEXIBILITY   Spend five minutes twice a day on seven of the stretching exercises described in Chapter 10.

AEROBIC FITNESS   Spend at least two weeks on each of the following levels and try to work out at least four times each week. To determine your target heart rate, subtract your age from 220 (to obtain your maximum rate), then compute 75 percent of that number. Or consult Cooper's Three-Mile Walking test at the beginning of the plan. Walking may be used as a target heart rate activity if you move at a brisk enough pace, although you may use any workout that sustains your target heart rate. Then finish your workout by walking at a more relaxed pace.

NUMBER OF MINUTES AT TARGET HEART RATE ACTIVITY	NUMBER OF MINUTES TO WALK
10	35
12	30
14	25
16	20
18	15
20	20

Spend a *minimum* of two weeks at each level.

Phase Three

FLEXIBILITY   Spend ten minutes, twice a day, incorporating all the stretching exercises described in Chapter 10. If you use running as your target heart rate activity, stretching becomes even more important because running causes the muscles along the back of the leg to shorten. Therefore, you may need to stretch more than the suggested amount of time.

AEROBIC FITNESS   Your entire workout should consist of target heart rate activity and you should aim for a minimum of four days a week. Begin your workout with five minutes of warm-up activity (walking, running in place, or very slow jogging) and end it with a five minute cool-down (walking, stretching). Spend four weeks at each level.

NUMBER OF MINUTES OF TARGET HEART RATE ACTIVITY

20-25
25-30
30-35
35-40
40-45
45-50
50-55
55-60

Spend a *minimum* of four weeks at each level.

▶▶ *Eating for Energy* ▶ ▶ ▶ ▶

The Energy Givers

Food is energy—if you eat the right kind. Unfortunately, most people don't understand what foods provide energy. To add to the problem, nutritionists have a different concept of nutrition than you or I do. To them food energy is the number of units of energy in a particular food. Units of energy are called kilocalories, hereafter called calories. A calorie is the amount of heat required to raise the temperature of one kilogram of water one degree centigrade—clear as mud. A more effective definition is given by Fergus M. Clydesdale, professor of Food Service and Nutrition at the University of Massachusetts. He says a calorie is "a unit of energy going into the body and supplying it with a certain amount of power, just as gas powers a car." A calorie itself is not actually fuel or food for the body. Instead, it is an abstract measurement, like an inch or a pound. One gram (about 1/28 of an ounce) of pure carbohydrate contains four calories. One gram of protein contains four calories. One gram of fat contains nine calories.

Since all foods are comprised of some combination of carbohydrates, fats, and proteins, a nutritionist or physiologist can calculate the number of calories in a particular food by determining the percentage of weight of the food that is carbohydrate, fat, and protein. So the next time you read a label of an eight-ounce fruit yogurt container that says there are 250 calories, you know that it was determined by a thorough analysis of the carbohydrate, fat, and protein content of the yogurt.

The quality and amounts of food that you eat have a direct bearing on your energy. Carbohydrates, fats, and proteins, assisted by minerals and vitamins, work together to help you achieve your maximum energy potential.

Carbohydrates

Carbohydrates are your body's most preferred nutrient. They are also the most maligned. Most of us think of them as the good-tasting treats from Grandma's kitchen that are too tempting to pass up. But they are also found in fruits, beets, onions, carrots, turnips, sweet potatoes, and other vegetables, as well as grains and grain products, such as breakfast cereals, pasta, and breads.

Carbohydrates are the easiest foods for your body to digest. Aside from providing energy, high-quality carbohydrate foods provide important minerals and vitamins, and oftentimes they come packaged with proteins.

When the carbohydrate stores in your body become inadequate, such as from prolonged, strenuous physical activity or starvation, the body can adjust and allow you to use fats and, infrequently, proteins to fill your energy needs. Unfortunately, the use of fats and proteins in place of carbohydrates is less-efficient and chemically more complex. The use of fats and proteins can continue for only a limited amount of time before other body functions begin to suffer.

Most carbohydrates come in the form of simple sugars or starches. When these carbohydrate foods are eaten, they are digested by your body and broken down into the simple sugars of *glucose, fructose,* and *galactose.* These carbohydrates may also be converted to *glycogen* for future use.

Glycogen is often called animal starch. It is stored in the liver or other tissues such as the muscles, as free or fixed glycogen. The free glycogen is released quickly for food energy whereas the fixed glycogen is released in a slower manner. Glycogen is used up quickly during exercise and starvation. Since most animals cannot store much glycogen, little of it is found in meat.

Cellulose is a carbohydrate but it's harder to digest than starches and sugars. It must be cooked to be digested. Even then, most of the cellulose remains undigested. Cellulose helps elimination by giving bulk to the digestive track. It comes from the seeds, leaves, stems, and roots of fruits.

There are four important points concerning carbohydrate energy:

1. Most of our energy from carbohydrates comes in the form of glucose.
2. Galactose and glucose need insulin to get across the cell membrane, fructose does not.
3. Starches are broken down more slowly by the body's digestive system.
4. Fructose is broken down, absorbed, and used more slowly than glucose and galactose.

These four concepts have important implications in energy utilization as will be shown in the next chapter.

Researchers agree that the optimum carbohydrate sources for energy are complex carbohydrates. The least desirable source is sucrose, since it floods the bloodstream with excessive glucose—but more on this later.

Complex carbohydrates allow for a steady stream of energy, releasing about two calories of energy per minute. This rate is ideally suited to the needs of your body.

A diet high in carbohydrates will give more stamina for heavy physical labor than will a diet high in protein, fats, or a combination of protein, fats, and carbohydrates. As far back as 1939, two Scandinavian physiologists, D.H. Christensen and O. Hansen, noted that the composition of a person's diet had a marked influence on how long he was able to continue heavy exercise. Diets rich in carbohydrates improved the exerciser's ability to continue exercising. Diets poor in carbohydrates, however, were associated with a reduced ability to exercise.

Almost 30 years later another group of Scandinavian physiologists determined that the relative composition of an exerciser's diet was closely related to the concentration of glycogen in the muscles. They further noted that exhaustion occurred when the muscle glycogen concentration was very low. A carbohydrate-rich diet increases the amount of muscle glycogen. This greater concentration of muscle glycogen delays the time when critically low levels of muscle glycogen are reached. Therefore, the length of time it takes for a person to become physically exhausted when exercising for long periods of time is increased. To go back to the automotive analogy, diets rich in carbohydrates act to increase the capacity of our fuel tanks, thus increasing our cruising range.

This technique of using carbohydrates for more energy is called carbohydrate loading, glycogen packing, or carbohydrate packing. Essentially, in carbohydrate loading the athlete attempts to increase his storage of glycogen before a performance or race. A seven-day regimen of glycogen loading might look like this:

Sunday:	Strenuous exercise	(depletion of glycogen stores)
Monday:	Moderate exercise	(very few carbohydrates)
Tuesday:	Moderate exercise	(very few carbohydrates)
Wednesday:	Light exercise	(plenty of carbohydrates)
Thursday:	Light exercise	(plenty of carbohydrates)
Friday:	Light exercise	(plenty of carbohydrates)
Saturday:	Competition	

The primary supply of carbohydrates should come from those foods listed in Table 11-1 (avoiding high amounts of pastry).

Carbohydrate loading causes you to first reduce your glycogen content and then you encourage your body to store an extra amount in the muscles—perhaps 10 percent. Caution should be taken, however, since carbohydrates tend to bind with water and some people experience a rather rapid weight gain (although it is water), and a feeling of sluggishness.

Just remember this important point: Carbohydrate loading works only when exercising two hours or more. It seems to have little value for the average tennis player, golfer, or jogger. But if you're going to split wood for two or three hours, bike, run a marathon, or work hard physically all day, it's good to know that carbohydrates are your best energy source.

It's important to note that we're suggesting changes in a relative proportion of one's diet during the days proceeding competition. Far too often, carbohydrate loading is interpreted to mean an excuse to go on a dietary binge. But that means trouble. Don't gorge yourself with cookies, donuts, pizza, and beer. If you overeat these foods you're going to feel like you've just finished a Thanksgiving or Christmas dinner. A relatively normal diet with somewhat reduced quantities of meat and dairy products and proportionately increased quantities of vegetables, fruits, and bread is best.

Table 11-1. Complex Carbohydrates

FRUCTOSE

Apples	Figs	Mangoes	Plums
Apricots	Gooseberries	Muskmelons	Pomegranates
Bananas	Grapefruit	Nectarines	Quinces
Blackberries	Grapes	Oranges	Raisins
Blueberries	Guava	Papayas	Raspberries
Breadfruit	Kumquats	Peaches	Strawberries
Cherries	Lemon juice	Pears	Tangerines
Cranberries	Loganberries	Persimmons	Watermelon
Dates	Lychees	Pineapple	

GRAINS

Barley	Cornmeal	Popcorn	Rye
Buckwheat	Oatmeal	Rice	Wheat

VEGETABLES

Artichokes	Carrots, raw	Legumes (dried)	Pumpkins
Asparagus	Cauliflower	Lentils	Radishes
Bamboo shoots	Celery	Lettuce	Rutabagas
Bean sprouts	Chives	Mustard greens	Squash
Beans, snap	Corn kernels	Okra	Sweet potatoes
(green & yellow)	Cucumbers	Onions	Swiss chard
Beans, lima	Eggplant	Parsley	Tapioca
Beans, pinto	Endive	Parsnips	Tomatoes
Beets	Garbanzos	Peas	Turnips
Broccoli	Garlic	Peppers	Water Chestnuts
Cabbage, raw	Leeks	Potatoes	

Fats

Fats have a bad reputation. Most people think that if they eat fats they'll get fat, but a certain amount of fat is essential if you expect to maintain a well-balanced energy diet.

Fats are actually a class of nutrients made up of fatty acids and glycerin (an organic alcohol). They are found in such foods as butter and other dairy products, fatty meats, fish, egg yolks, poultry, salad and cooking oils, margarine, chocolate, nuts, and peanut butter. Pound for pound, fats provide more usable energy (calories) than either carbohydrates or proteins. They also take longer to digest so you feel fuller after a meal or a snack that contains some fatty component.

Certain foods contain different chemical compounds, called fats or lipids. These include triglycerides, phospholipids, and cholesterol. The triglycerides are used in the body to provide energy, a function they share with the carbohydrates. The cholesterol and phospholipids, however, are used throughout the body for other cell functions. Consequently, the primary emphasis here will be on triglycerides.

Thirty to 50 percent of all the carbohydrates you eat with each meal are converted into triglycerides in the liver and then stored in the fat cells and later used as fatty acids for energy. Your body can store only small amounts of glycogen (carbohydrates). However, the average person can store up to 200 times as much energy in the form of fat. This difference is important when exercising for long periods of time or engaging in hard physical labor for many weeks.

During very light or moderate muscular exercise—walking, swimming, sailing, and easy jogging—energy is derived in almost equal amounts from your body's stores of carbohydrates and fats. In an all-out run, however, most of the energy comes from carbohydrates. That's because as the exercise becomes more and more intense, your body produces lactic acid. When lactic acid begins to appear in the blood some fatty acids are blocked, which means that your body must rely on carbohydrates for energy. The more intense the exercise, the more lactic acid; hence, fewer fatty acids are used.

When you exercise at more moderate levels your body works the other say. That is, if you run moderately or swim moderately for an hour or so, there is a significant shift in your body metabolism so that you start using more fatty acids and fewer carbohydrates. If you run for an hour or so, 90 percent of your energy may come from fats and 10 percent from carbohydrates.

This phenomenon of fat-utilization and of lactic acid blocking the fat has important energy implications. People who are unfit produce quite a bit of lactic acid at relatively low levels of exercise. Consequently, they use less fat for energy than do fit people. As they become fit, however, they produce less lactic acid and therefore burn more fat. The successful burning of fat helps to spare the carbohydrate—and they experience less fatigue.

The traditional approach to improving energy (as we discussed under carbohydrate energy) has been to attempt to enlarge the total amount of glycogen that the body can store. In other words, the body tries to create a large fuel storage tank. Interestingly, some researchers are also looking at how to spare the rate of glycogen used—how to improve the body's gas mileage. Most studies show that it's probably more important to slow the rate of glycogen release than it is to increase the total size of glycogen stores.

A runner's diet just before a run can have a profound influence upon the rate of glycogen used. Some runners who practice carbohydrate loading believe that extra carbohydrates should be eaten right up to the start of the race. That is not a good idea. Release of insulin into the blood following the eating of carbohydrates blocks the release of fatty acids from the fat tissue. Consequently, muscle glycogen and blood glucose are the only fuels potentially available for muscular contraction. During exercise, an increased rate of muscle glycogen use occurs and there's a rapid initial drop in blood glucose. If the exercise is continued, fatigue from muscle glycogen depletion occurs at a rate faster than normal. In a few people blood glucose continues to fall until hypoglycemia occurs. Hypoglycemia produces overpowering weariness, light-headedness, irritability, and occasional fainting. Those feelings occur when the blood glucose level falls to a point where the fuel supply to the brain becomes limited.

If the meal is eaten far enough in advance to allow complete digestion, the insulin levels will be normal, so the fatty acids are not blocked. In most cases, a meal three to six hours before prolonged exercise will allow adequate depletion. Most long exercise sessions are generally started in the mornings, so the most practical solution to the prerun feeding problem is to eat your last meal during the evening. That way you'll come to the start of the event with an empty stomach.

For example, let's say you plan a long hike one morning while on vacation. Eat a good, well balanced meal high in complex carbohydrates the night before. For breakfast, keep it light—perhaps a glass of orange juice and a piece of toast. Carry some fruit along the trail and eat that when you get hungry. After your hike, return to your normal eating habits. The key to eating before extended, strenuous exercise is to give your digestive system very little work to do from three to six hours before you begin. That way, you will improve your fuel economy.

Proteins

Proteins, present in all living tissues, make up vital parts of cells. They are the main constituents of muscles, nerves, glands, and many hormones. Protein molecules are large and are composed of many nitrogen-containing components called amino acids. Individual protein molecules may consist of several different amino acids. Before your body can use these proteins they must be broken down by the digestive system into their component amino acids. There are 21 amino acids, of which your body can manufacture 11 (called nonessential). The other 10, called essential amino acids, can be obtained only be eating the right foods.

Your body uses proteins to build and repair body tissues, and in emergency situations your body can oxidize proteins to meet energy needs. However, proteins can be used for energy only a short period of time, because while proteins are being oxidized for energy, the building and repairing process of body cells and tissues stops. When there is a lack of carbohydrates or fat your body must use protein for energy, but utilization of protein for food energy is far less efficient than using carbohydrates and fats. If your protein supply is not sufficient to offset the daily destruction of cells, your body actually begins to waste away.

Proteins are crucial, but are not required in large amounts. Meat, fish, eggs, and nuts are rich in complete protein, containing all the essential amino acids. Dry cereals, breads, and most fruits and vegetables contain lesser amounts of proteins. Additionally, these proteins do not contain all ten essential amino acids. These foods are good, but for most effective use by the body they should be combined with other protein fats to make them more effective (see Table 11-2).

It's important to get protein from a wide range of sources, particularly during periods of rapid growth and cell formation, as in adolescence, pregnancy, and convalescence. Many doctors thus prescribe high protein diets for pregnant women, and for individuals with diseases which have caused a high degree of cell destruction or damage.

Vitamins

Vitamins are not food energy sources per se (they don't provide calories), but vitamins are a very important energy source, making it possible for us to use appropriately the food we eat. They provide for chemical control of your body functions and play an important role in energy production, normal growth, resistance to infection, and general health. Most vitamins act as catalysts that initiate or speed up the rate of chemical reactions. Life cannot continue without these biochemical catalysts.

Nevertheless, vitamins cannot catalyze anything on their own. They must first combine with substances called apoenzymes, which are manufactured within each individual cell. When a cell is making apoenzymes at its maximum speed, and they are combining with vitamins as fast as they are made, the cell is said to be saturated with that particular vitamin. Once the whole body is saturated, any excess vitamins are either stored or circulated in the bloodstream.

Table 11-2. Protein Foods

ANIMAL PRODUCTS

Beef	Duck	Fish	Pork
Cheese	Eggs	Milk	Turkey
Chicken			

GRAINS

Brown Rice	Corn	Oats	Rice

LEGUMES

Garbanzo Beans	Lima Beans	Peas	Soybean Flour
Kidney Beans	Mung Beans	Soy Sprouts	Soybeans

NUTS AND SEEDS

Cashews	Peanuts

VEGETARIAN DISHES*

Barley and yogurt soup	Middle Eastern hummus
Bean or pea curry on rice	(sesame and chick-peas)
Blended dip of garbanzos,	Milk in legume soups
sesame, lemon, garlic, oil	Pasta with milk or cheese
Bread made with milk or cheese	Pea soup and toast
Breads with added seed meals	Rice and milk pudding
Breads with sesame or	Rice-bean casserole
sunflower seed spread	Rice-cheese casserole
Cereal with milk	Rice with sesame seeds
Cheese sandwiches	Roasted seeds—soybean snack
Cheese sauce for garbanzo beans	Sesame salt on legume dish
Corn-soy bread	Sesame seeds in bean soups and
Corn tortillas and beans	casseroles
Legume soup with bread	Sunflower seeds and peanuts
Lentil curry on rice	Wheat berries with cheese sauce
Macaroni and cheese	Wheat bread with baked beans
	Wheat-soy bread

SOURCE: Based on Frances Lappe's *Diet for a Small Planet*, New York, Ballantine.

* These dishes show how you can combine nonmeat protein foods (those not containing all ten essential amino acids) to make a complete protein dish.

Most plants manufacture the vitamins they need. For the most part, your body can't do that. You must get your vitamins from the foods you eat. The highest sources of vitamins are meats; fruits; vegetables; milk; eggs; fish; and certain cereals. Vitamin deficiencies can result in night blindness, poor bone and tooth formation, scurvy, stunted growth, lack of vitality, poor condition of skin and mucous membranes, and a loss of appetite and weight.

When many people talk about nutrition they think only of vitamins. They faithfully study the chart on the side of the cereal boxes to see whether they're getting their vitamins. But if you ate nothing but bowls of cereal every day for the rest of your life and nothing else, you probably wouldn't live very long, even if you thought you were getting enough vitamins. That's because you're simply getting vitamins and carbohydrates, and not an adequate amount of protein, selected minerals, and other essential vitamins.

There is a tremendous controversy regarding how much of each vitamin is needed by Americans. On one side of the coin, the traditional medical establishment advocates the United States government recommended daily allowance (RDA) on vitamins. (See Table 11-3.) On the other side of the coin, two famous biochemists, Dr. Linus Pauling and Roger Williams, recommend megavitamins. However, the role of vitamins in building energy is very cloudy. Researchers just don't know. Most of the studies show that supplementing an already well-balanced diet will not produce an increase in energy. But most of these studies have been conducted over relatively short periods of time. We don't know what effect vitamin supplementation has over a 10-, 15-, or 20-year period of time.

Research however, has demonstrated that certain people need extra vitamins. Heavy drinkers, for example, are often deficient in many of the B vitamins. Very heavy drinkers have an even more serious problem: After six or seven drinks a day over a two-week period of time they begin to suffer from starvation no matter how much they eat and no matter how well balanced their diet is. Under conditions of alcohol abuse, the small intestine pours out fluids and flushes food from the body before vitamins and minerals can be absorbed.

Heavy smokers often suffer depletion of vitamin C. Additionally, women using a birth control pill seem to have difficulty securing enough of the B vitamins and vitamin C.

We cannot assume that if a little of a vitamin is good for you, a lot is even better. When cells are vitamin saturated, additional vitamins are worthless. Consequently, I advise experimentation.

My own recommendation is to make sure that you get your RDA. If you decide to go to the megadoses I would suggest that you discuss this with your physician. (Note: I also suggested that you get as many of your vitamins as possible from fresh fruits and vegetables, either raw or steamed. If you must cook them, cook lightly and try to save the juice. Also choose whole grain breads and cereals rather than refined ones, and select brown rice instead of white. Finally, eat a wide variety of foods. As for meat, try seafood and fowl in place of pork and beef.)

Table 11-3. U.S. Recommended Daily Allowances (RDA) of Vitamins and Minerals

KEY

1 microgram (mcg.)	=	1/1000 of a milligram = 1 gamma
1,000 micrograms	=	1 milligram (mg.)
1,000 milligrams	=	1 gram (g.)
1,000 grams	=	1 kilogram (kg.)

VITAMIN	U.S. RDA
A	5,000 International Units (IU)
D	200-400 IU (5-10 mcg.)
E	15 IU Men (10 mg.); 12 IU Women (8 mg.)
K	70-140 mcg.
B$_1$ Thiamine	1.4 mg. Men; 1 mg. Women
B$_2$ Riboflavin	1.6 mg. Men; 1.2 mg. Women
B$_3$ Niacin	18 mg. Men; 13 mg. Women
B$_5$ Pantothenic Acid	4-7 mg.
B$_6$ Pyridoxine	2.2 mg. Men; 2 mg. Women
Biotin	1.3 mg.
Folacin	1.4 mg.
B$_{12}$ Cyanocabalamin	3 mcg.
C	60 mg.

MINERAL	U.S. RDA
Calcium	800 mg.
Magnesium	350 mg. Men; 300 mg. Women
Phosphorus	800 mg.
Potassium	1,875-5,625 mg.
Sodium	1,100-3,300 mg.
Sulfur	...

TRACE MINERAL	U.S. RDA
Chromium	.05-.2 mg.
Copper	2-3 mg.
Fluorine	...
Iodine	150 mcg.
Iron	18 mg.
Manganese	2.5-5 mg.
Selenium	...
Zinc	15 mg.

Minerals

Minerals are unique, inorganic chemical substances that play an important part in regulating body functions. They are essential to the structure of bones and other body tissues, and vital to energy.

Minerals are part of the cell membrane, cell nucleus, and other cell structures—such as the mitochondria, the powerhouse of the cell. This powerhouse converts food nutrients to energy. For example, selected minerals help break down glucose, fatty acids, and amino acids into energy. All other minerals build up the glucose, fatty acids, and amino acids into glycogen, fats, and proteins respectively. Minerals also serve as important parts of the structure of various hormones, enzymes, and other substances that help to regulate the chemical reactions within cells.

For years nutritionists have emphasized the major minerals: calcium, magnesium, phosphorus, potassium, sodium, and sulfur. These have been considered the essential nutrients. More recently the trace elements or minerals have been brought to the fore. Work begun by Dr. Henry A. Schroeder, professor emeritus at Dartmouth Medical School, has demonstrated that trace elements, although present in minute amounts, are essential for normal metabolism. They include chromium, copper, fluorine, iodine, iron, manganese, selenium, zinc, and a few others.

According to Schroeder's thesis, unlike vitamins, which are synthesized by plants and animals, minerals—of equal or even greater importance— must come from the outside, and failure to include them in our diets can lead to trouble.

Schroeder notes that those elements that occur in amounts less than 0.01 percent of the human body are trace elements. While this definition is narrow and restrictive, research demonstrates that they are important for our health and maximum personal energy.

The Energy Robbers 12 ►►

Just as some foods give energy, other foods steal energy. These foods have the potential to undo some or all of the good expected from the energy givers. Commonly called "junk foods", these are high in calories and low in nutrients. They contain excessive amounts of one or more of the following: sugar, fat, salt, and caffeine.

Your body has an amazing ability to tolerate abuse, by making many adjustments to help you survive and maintain homeostasis—the balance within the body to maintain health and life. But consuming too much sugar, fats, salt, and caffeine, as many Americans do, causes personal energy levels to decline. As much as you don't want to admit it, you can't have maximum personal energy while living on hamburgers, cokes, milkshakes, french fries, doughnuts, and other deep-fried concoctions, as well as candy, coffee, pretzels, cakes, and cream-filled "goodies." They're all "baddies" for your energy.

I know what you might be thinking: runners who have won both the Boston and New York Marathons, literally pig out on coffee, soda, candy bars, doughnuts, ice cream, and mayonnaise. Yet they have energy to burn. First, understand one very important fact: People like this are biologically special. You cannot compare yourself to them. While they might get away with a certain pattern of eating, it does not logically follow that you can do the same thing—unless you have been blessed with their physical attributes.

Second, if it were possible for one marathoner to compete against himself—that is, one marathoner on a good diet versus the same marathoner on a bad diet—I'd put my money on the good-eating marathoner.

Third, most premier marathoners are in their late twenties and early thirties. Many people don't feel tired at this point in their life. It's usually after eating a jitterbug diet for 30 years that people start to fall apart and feel tired.

Fourth, marathoners do follow several other high-energy living patterns. They run, stretch, practice relaxation techniques, don't smoke, and use few drugs. As a result, they don't feel the energy drain until later in life.

You simply can't cozy up to junk foods and still achieve your maximum personal energy. There are many reasons why. To start with, take a look at sugar, a major "junk" ingredient, to see how it saps energy.

Sugar

While "just a spoonful of sugar" may not harm your energy levels, eating 100 to 120 pounds a year (as the average American does) is energy suicide. That's the entire sugar jar or 20 teaspoons a day. To compound the problem, the average American eats only 5 pounds of fruit, vegetables, and cereal products for every pound of sugar. In 1909, the average was 10 pounds of the wholesome stuff for every pound of sugar. Sugar may give a temporary lift (20 minutes), but later in the day and over the long haul, it's counterproductive to your energy level.

Speed of Digestion and Insulin Reaction

Sucrose is ultimately broken down into glucose and fructose for energy. As glucose, it gets into your bloodstream very quickly and then requires insulin to get into your cells. The speed of digestion, the insulin requirement, and the amount of sugar eaten by the average American causes a severe lack of energy.

Your body's blood sugar level is monitored by both the hypothalamus in the brain and the pancreas. When the blood sugar level falls too low (usually if you haven't eaten for several hours), glucose is released from the liver and/or the fat stores are activated. When your blood sugar level goes too high, insulin is secreted by the pancreas to help speed the glucose into the cells, thereby reducing the blood glucose levels.

Certain people, however, seem to have difficulty in handling single sugars well—especially large quantities of single sugars. These individuals experience varying degrees of fatigue, blurred vision, a drunken gait, slurred speech, nausea, sudden changes in mood such as depression, crying, and hostility.

Scientists have not been able to pinpoint the exact cause for this condition. In fact, some doctors believe the condition is a figment of their patient's imagination. However, the fatigue may be caused by hypoglycemia or hyperosmolality. Work done by Dr. William J. Hudspeth, associate professor, Department of Psychiatry and Behavioral Science at the University of Nevada School of Medicine in Reno, demonstrates these potential problems quite nicely. His research also demonstrates why some doctors have missed the diagnosis of sugar metabolism problems.

In hypoglycemia too much insulin is secreted, forcing an excessive amount of glucose into the cells and, thereby, reducing blood glucose levels to very low levels. The result is fatigue, depression, dizziness. This condition is easy to recognize since the patient will have low blood sugar levels.

However, some patients demonstrate these same symptoms but do not have low blood sugar levels. Their condition may be hyperosmolality. In hyperosmolality an excessive amount of insulin is secreted, wreaking havoc on the body. And the one part that seems most affected by the insulin is the brain. According to Hudspeth, "Too much insulin can cause brain cells to absorb more than the usual number of electrolytes (ions that circulate in the blood) and to swell with water." Consequently, the patient exhibits characteristics similar to hypoglycemia. This condition, however, can be detected only by the glucose tolerance test, EEGs (brain wave patterns), and actual glucose and insulin levels. That's why some doctors have missed the patient's problem.

The bottom line is that fatigue can be caused by a poor diet. For some people the problem may be too much blood sugar, for others it may be too much insulin, but for both the cause is the same—eating too much sugar.

The treatment for both conditions is also the same. According to Hudspeth, "Keep excessive insulin reactions down by sticking to a diet that is low in refined carbohydrates (natural sources are all right) and low in protein, and by reducing stress."

Athletes must also be very much aware of the sugar/insulin reaction. Dr. David Costill of Ball State University's Human Performance Laboratory has noted that insulin accelerates the removal of glucose from the blood. Exercise does the same thing—even if insulin is absent. Therefore, an athlete who eats a lot of sugar at the start of a race or before the event is headed for trouble. The combination of high insulin secretion and the muscular activity of running causes the glucose to be removed from the blood at a rate faster than either the intestines or the liver can handle efficiently. The exerciser's muscles are suddenly deprived of their most important source of fuel—blood glucose, so the body must rely on its next most important source—muscle glycogen. Glycogen is not converted nearly as quickly as glucose, so performance is significantly impaired.

Everything I've talked about up to this point focuses on sucrose. Little is known about what happens when a person eats large amounts of milk or fruit sugar—lactose or fructose. Fructose may be somewhat better than sucrose because it is absorbed more slowly and does not need insulin to pass into the cells. Consequently, blood sugar may not drop as fast. The same is true of honey, which is high in fructose. Since fructose breaks down slowly during metabolism, it does not overload the pancreas and cause it to release more insulin.

As you will recall from the previous chapter, I also mentioned that the complex carbohydrates are absorbed more slowly and are released into the bloodstream at about two calories per minute. This steady stream of energy is perfect for your body. Consequently, if you are going to eat before strenuous exercise, it would be far better to eat a diet high in complex carbohydrates rather than simple sugars. Fructose may also be a satisfactory replacement.

The Amount Eaten

The problem with sugar (or sucrose) is the amount eaten, rather than sucrose itself. If people ate only a few pounds of sugar a year, or a fraction of an ounce a day, the above discussion would not apply; but the average American eats about 2 to 2 1/2 pounds of sugar a week, or 500 to 750 calories a day of pure sugar. This is too much. It amounts to 20 to 25 percent of total caloric intake.

A diet high in sucrose tends to be low in other basic nutrients—especially the B vitamins and several essential minerals, because most sugar comes highly refined and stripped of any potential of giving a positive contribution to your energy. The best diet includes many natural vegetables and grain products (complex carbohydrates) and small amounts of simple sugars.

Fats

Fats can be a source of energy, but like everything else in this chapter, they are a double-edged sword. Too much can cause problems.

According to many scientists, fats can steal energy for several reasons. First, fats can actually suffocate tissues by depriving them of oxygen. Both saturated and unsaturated fats form a fatty film around the red blood cells and platelets in the blood, causing the cells and platelets to stick together. This sludging causes the red blood cells to carry less oxygen and even plug tiny blood vessels (capillaries). When capillaries get blocked, the watery part of the blood is forced through the capillary walls causing edema—which reduces the amount of oxygen available to the cells. Some experts say this plugging can affect 5 to 20 percent of your body tissue. Smoking after a heavy, fatty meal compounds the problem. The carbon monoxide in the smoke crowds out even more oxygen, hence less oxygen gets to the tissues.

Second, a high fat diet may raise cholesterol levels. This cholesterol tends to deposit on the lining of the arteries. When these linings are occluded, less oxygen gets to the heart and you become a prime candidate for heart disease.

Third, fats steal energy through the condition of ketosis. A high-fat, high-protein, low-carbohydrate diet is often used to achieve weight loss, but many dieters develop unbelievable fatigue. Their diet is largely fat, so the sugar in the blood is burned off rapidly, forcing the body to depend on fat reserves for energy. The fatty acids derived from the fat reserve burn inefficiently. As a result, they produce acid metabolites called ketones. Doctors call this ketone increase ketosis.

In ketosis your metabolism resembles that of a diabetic. It is a dangerous condition because the brain is partially starved by the absence of glucose. Glucose is the brain's only source of food, and fatty acids cannot be converted to glucose. Furthermore, ketones are acidic. They may actually change your blood pH. A highly acid blood also makes it hard for the body and brain to function properly. A change in blood Ph will produce tremendous fatigue, since a fine balance must be kept. If the blood becomes acidic enough, the resulting ketosis shock may be fatal.

Finally, it has been shown that an excessive amount of fatty acids in the bloodstream can cause irregular heartbeats and possibly present problems for the liver.

The conclusion: a high-protein, high-fat, low-carbohydrate diet causes the dieter to feel whipped most of the time. My advice: avoid it.

Salt

When we discuss salt, we need to make the distinction between sodium and sodium chloride. Sodium is a trace mineral found naturally in many foods. A body needs regular, small amounts of sodium. Sodium chloride, however, is a chemically manufactured salt commonly referred to as table salt.

Americans eat more table salt (consequently more sodium) than their bodies need. The average person probably needs no more than a gram a day. Yet, many Americans eat 8 to 15 grams per day. They believe salt makes everything taste better. But it doesn't. Salt has a taste of its own. People who use it are enjoying the taste of the table salt, not the fruit, vegetable, or meat.

Yet, the typical American palate responds to any and all foods with one four-word phrase, "It needs more salt."

Unfortunately, too much sodium may be a precipitator of hypertension or high blood pressure. In sodium-sensitive people, high blood pressure is one of the biggest causes for fatigue in this country. So, if you have fatigue and don't know what your blood pressure is, have your doctor check it for you. High blood pressure may cause fatigue because of a feedback mechanism. When blood pressure rises, your body assumes you need rest to drop the pressure. So, selected receptors signal you to be tired. When you rest, your blood pressure drops.

Some cardiologists claim that if we eliminated salt from the American diet there would be no high blood pressure in the U.S.A. Other experts claim the jury is still out. But one thing is clear: cultures around the world that eat little salt—Eskimos, Australians, Aborigines, and Panamanian Indians—have very low rates of high blood pressure, while people like the Northern Japanese, who eat 35 or more grams of salt a day, have unbelievably high rates of hypertension—four persons out of ten. Also, when a person eats a diet low in salt after having high blood pressure, the blood pressure usually drops significantly.

Some people worry they will get too little salt, but there is absolutely no cause for concern. Practically everything you eat contains some salt. The average American's largest supply of salt (other than that sprinkled on food) comes from pork, ham, and bacon. One serving of ham provides as much as two grams of salt, so replacing salt naturally is not difficult. Most cheeses also have a high level of salt and are a good, natural way for replacing salt. Fruits generally have a low salt content, but the banana stands above all others as a good supply of salt. Most vegetables do not contain a great deal of salt either, but endive greens, lettuce, potatoes, and spinach offer higher amounts of salt than other vegetables. In addition, many foods are little else than carriers of salt. These include olives, pickles, relishes, luncheon meats, and dried beef. If you are concerned about not getting enough salt due to an excess of sweating and/or of high-humidity exercise, choosing foods from Table 12-1 will help replace that salt.

At one time salt tablets were recommended for people who sweated a great deal, but no more. High salt intake is not necessary except for those who exercise in an extremely hot environment over a long period of time, and the use of salt tablets is not recommended at all. There are exceptions, but as a general rule you can assume that the less salt you eat, the better off you will be. If you feel you need extra salt, get it from the natural, wholesome foods on the list, (marked by an asterisk), rather than by salting foods.

Table 12-1. High-Salt Foods

All canned and frozen foods	Frankfurters and sausages	Pickles
Bacon	Garlic salt	Pretzels
Beets*	Gravy	Relishes
Bouillon cubes	Ham	Salt pork
Canned meats	Kale*	Salted butter
Canned soups or stews	Ketchup	Salted, dried, and
Carrots*	Luncheon meats	smoked fish and meats
Caviar	Meat sauces	Salted nuts
Celery salt	Milk*	Salted popcorn
Cheese*	Mustard	Salted margarine
Chili sauce	Mustard greens*	Shellfish
Commercial salad dressings	Olives	Soy sauce
Commercially made:	Onion salt	Spinach*
breads, rolls, crackers	Organ meats	Tenderizers
Dandelion greens*	Pickled foods (sauerkraut)	Worcestershire sauce

*Foods with naturally high content of salt.

Caffeine

While there may be nothing better than the smell of coffee perking on the stove, drinking it can seriously affect your supply of energy. Most people who drink coffee think it has a stimulating effect. Indeed, laboratory experiments indicate that coffee increases mental alertness, speeds reaction time, and actually helps people think more clearly.

Along with these apparent benefits, caffeine may improve your performance in endurance events such as marathon running. It has been shown that caffeine promotes an increased release of fatty acids from the fatty tissues. That means muscle glycogen will be spared, thus slowing the onset of fatigue. Such information indicates a cup of coffee may be a great way to stay alert, run a better marathon, or provide you with energy.

Before jumping to conclusions, however, consider the other side of the research. The culprit in coffee is caffeine. When even small amounts of this substance enter your body, it begins to create some changes. After the initial perk to your cardiovascular system, caffeine goes to work on your muscles. They react to this chemical by tensing up. In fact, even three to five hours after your last cup of coffee, your metabolism can remain increased from 10 to 25 percent. That means you are using more energy even though you may not be working any harder than normal. The cumulative effect contributes to that "tired, worn-out" feeling at the end of the day.

Still another energy-related problem is insomnia. The primary ingredient in over-the-counter "pep pills" is caffeine. College students quickly discover that a few cups of strong, black coffee will help them stay up all night to study for an exam. A student rationalizes this practice by planning to get more sleep the next day. An executive, however, who drinks up to eight cups of coffee through the day and suffers with sleeplessness that night still has to get up for work the next day—feeling very tired. It's a pattern of living that's devastating to your energy supply: the coffee increases your metabolism, constantly picking you up throughout the day then dropping you in a tired heap throughout the evening, only to keep you up all night. Additionally, some scientists report that caffeine may influence certain brain receptors in such a way that they block the brain's own tranquilizing hormone. The result is increased anxiety.

Of course, different people handle caffeine in different ways. Some people drink large amounts of coffee and still don't experience skipped heartbeat, anxiety, insomnia, and the jitters. Others take one cup of coffee and are so hyped up that they swear off coffee for the rest of their lives. If you drink coffee, recollect how many cups it used to take to stimulate you. If at one time one cup seemed to perk you up and now it takes two or more, you can conclude that your body is adapting to the amount of caffeine.

Does this mean you need to give up coffee entirely in your quest for more energy? Eventually, that might be a good goal. But a more sensible approach right now would be to try to cut back a little. If you are drinking ten cups of coffee a day, see if you can reduce that to five or six cups. Once you notice the benefits of getting by with a little less caffeine, you will probably become more encouraged to cut back even a little more. If you can limit your daily intake of coffee to three cups or less, and make sure you aren't getting more from other sources, that amount of caffeine may not seriously affect your energy level.

At the same time, be more aware of the other sources of caffeine such as tea, cocoa, or colas. A cup of tea contains between 60 to 75 mg. of caffeine depending upon whether you're using instant, leaf, or bag tea. Cocoa contains up to 50 mg. of caffeine and many cola drinks contain anywhere between 40 to 60 mg.

Americans consume excessive amounts of caffeine beginning at a very early age. Children eat or drink huge quantities of caffeine from soft drinks, candy bars, and colas. Thus a young child may weigh only 40 to 50 pounds and consume the caffeine equivalent for his body weight of an adult drinking eight cups of coffee each day. If your child is irritable, nervous, or doesn't sleep well, it's very likely that caffeine is the culprit. The excessive energy your child has may be symptomatic of too much caffeine. On the other hand, some research suggests that children may have an opposite response to caffeine—lethargy. Regardless, keep the caffeine content low with young children. Otherwise, it'll eventually wipe them out.

Dieting

The less said about dieting the better. Dieting is the pits when it comes to energy. Most dieters skip meals—breakfast in particular. Then they have a mid-morning snack or wait until noon to eat. This means that they probably have gone 15 hours or more without any food. No wonder that by 11:00 a.m. or so they feel famished, irritable—and tired. Low blood sugar might be the cause, or it might just be the lack of carbohydrates. Unfortunately, at this time most people have a sweet roll and coffee. And they may put a little cream and some sugar in the coffee. The result is a temporary lift and then a big letdown, all because of the exhausting combination of fat, sugar, and caffeine, a deadly triad. To break this cycle, eat a decent breakfast, or at coffee break time eat some fresh fruit, vegetables, or cheese.

Diets also tend to restrict the eating of certain foods—carbohydrates in particular. You need carbohydrates for higher energy levels. The cutting out of other foods may short-change you on vitamins and minerals.

Most dieters are tired all the time. The only thing that keeps them going and gives them a lift is seeing fewer pounds on the scale and wearing smaller-sized clothing. Unfortunately, 90 to 95 percent of all diets fail. They do so because people cannot fight the overwhelming fatigue that's associated with dieting, and also the basic human drive for food.

Eating is okay—honest. Just don't skip meals, make sure you eat the right balance of energy givers, and cut back on the energy robbers.

A Plan for Eating for Energy

Traditionally, nutritionists based their recommendations for eating on the four basic food groups (milk, meat, bread-cereal, and vegetable-fruit), which were introduced in the mid 1950s in an effort to translate the many nutrient recommendations into simple food choices. In the *Eating for Energy Plan,* those four basic food groups have been expanded to six so that you will be certain to enjoy a complete and nutritious diet.

The *Eating for Energy Plan* is low in processed and refined foods and high in fresh and frozen fruits and vegetables. It is high in complex carbohydrates and low in fat. Virtually all sugar and salt have been eliminated from your regular eating pattern, though now and then you may feel free to dip into your passion food barrel you once subsisted on.

Work your way into this diet plan gradually, rather than trying to change your eating habits "cold turkey." As your nutrition improves, you'll note a significant increase in your energy level.

IMPORTANT NOTE: Whenever you are given a choice of several options and are allowed a certain amount weekly or monthly, make sure you follow the recommended number of servings. For example, if you are allowed a total of 2 to 3 servings of the various meats listed, that does not mean 2 to 3 servings of herring, 2 to 3 servings of mackerel, 2 to 3 servings of salmon, etc. If you have one serving of herring, one serving of mackerel, and one serving of salmon throughout the week, that is your limit for that week. The same holds true for all options throughout the plan.

A nutrition purist might criticize our inclusion of selected foods 1-3 times per week (foods that contain sugar, salt, and saturated fats). This plan, however, takes into consideration that maintaining a prudent, energy-giving diet is sometimes difficult in our society. It is designed to help a person select the best possible foods from a variety of choices. Also, you must remember that few foods are entirely good or bad. Milk is a nutritious beverage, yet contains high levels of saturated fats. Rather than cut milk out of your diet entirely, this plan recommends a limit to the amount of whole milk you drink.

A Plan for Eating for Energy

Servings Per Day	Food Group	Foods Which May Be Eaten Anytime	Foods Which May Be Eaten 2-3 Times a Week	Foods Which May Be Eaten Once a Week	Foods Which May Be Eaten Once a Month
3-5	**Group 1 Vegetables.** Asparagus, broccoli, carrots, chicory, collards, corn, cucumbers, eggplant, green peas, kale, mustard greens, onions, parsnips, parsley, potatoes, pumpkins, rutabagas, spinach, squash, string beans, sweet potatoes, wax beans, and white turnips.	All fresh and frozen vegetables such as those listed on the left.	Salted vegetable juices, i.e., V-8 juice, or salted canned soups and vegetables.	Salted vegetable juices, i.e., V-8 juice, or salted canned soups and vegetables. May have 2-3 servings a week total.	French fries, olives, and pickles.
2-4	**Group 2 Fruits.** Apples, bananas, berries, cabbage, cantaloupe, figs, grapefruit, grapes, lemons, limes, mangoes, oranges, papayas, peaches, pears, pineapples, plums, prunes, raisins and tomatoes. Juices are permitted.	All frozen and fresh citrus fruits, cabbage, and salad greens. Juices are also permitted.	Sweetened berry, lemons, grapefruit, orange, etc., juices.	Salted tomato juice.	
2	**Group 3 Milk and milk products.**	Buttermilk, farmer or pot cheese, low-fat cottage cheese, low-fat milk with 1% milk fat, skim milk, and ricotta skim milk	Frozen low-fat yogurt, low-fat milk with 2% milk fat, low-fat (2%) yogurt plain or sweetened, and regular cottage cheese (4% milk fat).	Hard cheese: blue, brick, camembert, cheddar (note: part-skim mozzarella and part-skim ricotta are preferable but still rich in fat), ice milk, processed cheese, whole milk, and whole milk yogurt.	Ice cream.

A Plan for Eating for Energy

Servings Per Day	Food Group	Foods Which May Be Eaten Anytime	Foods Which May Be Eaten 2-3 Times a Week	Foods Which May Be Eaten Once a Week	Foods Which May Be Eaten Once a Month
2 (about 4 oz. total)	**Group 4 Meats, poultry, fish, dried beans, rice, lentils, soybeans, peas, nuts, peanut butter, and eggs.**	Chicken or turkey (no skin). Fish such as cod, flounder, haddock, halibut, perch, pollock, rockfish, shellfish (except shrimp), sole, tuna (water-packed), egg whites, rice, and lentils.	Fish such as herring, mackerel, salmon, sardines, shrimp, and tuna (oil-packed). Red meat such as flank steak, ham, leg of lamb, plate beef, round steak, rump roast, sirloin steak, veal, soybeans, and peanut butter.	Deep-fried and breaded fish and poultry, ground beef, liver, pork loin, spareribs, untrimmed meats, egg yolks or whole eggs.	Bacon, corned beef, hot dogs, salami, sausage, luncheon meats, i.e., bologna, and liverwurst.
4	**Group 5 Whole grain breads and cereals.**	Barley, bread and rolls (whole grain), bulghur, oatmeal, pasta, whole grain cereal (except granola).	Unsweetened granola cereals.	Sweetened granola and traditional packaged cereals.	Pre-sweetened cereals and white bread.
In moderation	**Group 6 Vegetable oils and fats.**	Margarines made with non-hydrogenated soybean oil	Mayonnaise, salad oils, and soft tub margarines.	Butter, cream, cream cheese, and sour cream.	Lard.
	Snack Foods			Angel food cake, animal crackers, fig bars, gingerbread, gingersnaps, popcorn (with small amounts of salt and butter), and sherbet.	Chocolate, coconut, commercial pies, pastries, donuts, potato chips and soda pop.

▶ ▶ *Slimming for Energy* ▶ ▶

Fat and Where It's At ▸**13**▸▸

I f you were to identify people you know who are dynamos of energy, you would probably notice that most are slim and trim. That in itself should tell you something about the relationship between energy and obesity. People who have an overabundance of body fat generally do not have the energy of those who have only a small percentage of body fat.

Fat, as you learned in Chapter 11, is important and functional. It acts as your energy storehouse. This stored fat gives you energy for the long run, or for chopping wood, walking long distances, playing tennis for several hours, or digging a ditch all day long. That is the good news of fat. The bad news is that too much fat can rob you of energy.

Fat as an Energy Robber

The fat cells of your body are your fuel storage tanks. When you burn off fewer calories through activity than your body takes in, you convert these extra calories into fat. To illustrate this point, suppose that you eat 2,400 calories worth of food during a 24-hour period, and your level of activity is such that you burn off exactly 2,400 calories as you work, sleep, and play your way through the day. Supply and demand are equal. Your body neither calls on reserves to make up an energy deficit, nor does it deposit extra calories in the form of fat. You are maintaining your weight. However, if you consume 2,400 calories and burn off only 2,300 of them, your body will convert those 100 unnecessary calories of food into fat and "store" it until it is needed for energy.

One pound of fat is the equivalent of 3,500 unnecessary calories. Whether these calories are eaten in the form of sirloin steak, ice cream, or raw carrots makes no difference. A calorie is a calorie. With this in mind, you can see that if you eat 100 calories a day more than you burn off through physical activity, at the end of 35 days, you'll have gained a pound. If you continue at the same rate, you'll be ten pounds heavier at the end of the year.

Fat is okay, provided it does not exceed 19 percent (men) or 23 percent (women) of your overall weight. When it exceeds that range it puts a drain on your energy levels.

When excess fat is put on, there is more body tissue to take care of. Your skeletal and muscle systems are under strain to support the additional lard. Your heart and lungs must work harder in order to assist your muscles in moving all the fat around. The extra fat causes your resting and working heart rate to be higher. For many people it may be 10 to 30 beats higher for any task, and the heart may beat 14,000 to 42,000 more times per day.

The extra fat problem, unfortunately, goes beyond heart beats and tired muscles and bones. Excess fat can cause problems for the arteries themselves. The buildup of fat in the vessels is energy-robbing. While fat is constantly transported throughout your blood vessels to be deposited in the fat cells of your body, too much fat heightens the possibility that the walls of your arteries will accumulate the fat, thus restricting the blood flow in the artery. It's much like an old pipe that is starting to clog up with rust and mineral deposits.

The clogging of the arteries slows the blood supply to the muscles, organs, and other tissues. As a result the body becomes less efficient. The clogging also causes the blood vessels to lose their elasticity or flexibility. The walls tear and thicken so that the vessels are narrowed even more. The blood must be pushed with greater force to continue circulation. The heart is forced to work harder. Blood pressure increases. Sometimes small vessels are entirely blocked and circulation to these peripheral areas of the body is cut off. Thus some people experience poor circulation and "cold feet." But the feet and hands are not the only places where these vessels are located. They are also found in the heart, the brain, and in various other organs. The result is less efficiency and more fatigue.

As the fatty deposits continue to accumulate, and the loss of flexibility in the arteries becomes more significant, the circulatory system gets even more sluggish. The blood vessels become less elastic and breathing becomes more shallow. In short, cardiovascular fitness drops and early fatigue sets in. With less exercise there is a further decrease in cardiovascular fitness. A vicious cycle ensues: less work, less fitness, more fatigue, less work. Soon people become so unfit that they avoid exercise at all costs. They simply don't have the stamina to keep it up any longer.

A quick review shows there are many physiological energy-draining syndromes that result from being too fat:

1. Muscles and bones must labor under great strain.
2. Heart and lungs must work harder to assist muscles.
3. Blood pressure increases, causing physical fatigue.
4. Blood vessels become less elastic, further decreasing circulation.
5. Fatty deposits build up on blood vessel linings.

Fat and Emotional Fatigue

Poor self-concept and lousy interpersonal relationships can lead to the blues. The blues are soon followed by despondency, depression, and ultimately, fatigue. Psychologists tell us that self-esteem is important in determining your overall energy levels. In our society, having an expanding waistline, or wide hips, or unattractive thighs falls short of our definition of beauty. Thus, you end up despising your body, yourself, and the world.

The stress brought on by this attitude is vicious. Stress, or depression, causes overeating in those people who have learned to eat under stressful conditions. The overeating causes them to consume more calories than they burn off. An increase in fatness ensues. With an increase in fatness people become less active, which results in no natural outlet for their stress. Thereby, a "catch-22" syndrome is set in motion.

Additionally, those who carry too much body fat are often tagged with the incorrect term "lazy." They're far from lazy. These poor, tired individuals are struggling through life with a distinct, energy-robbing burden. They're not lazy, just overloaded psychologically and physically, and consequently they're worn out.

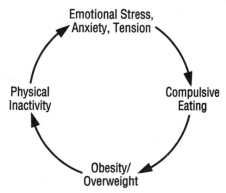

Fat and Weight

You may have noticed that I never mention being overweight. Instead, I refer to a condition of obesity, or too much body fat. This is an important distinction, and one you need to understand to discuss the concept of slimming to increase energy. Let me begin by making two apparently contradictory statements:

A person can be underweight, yet obese.

A person can be overweight and not obese.

Sounds confusing, doesn't it? That's because for so long we have been slaves to the scales and the height/weight charts; we have failed to understand the concept of lean body tissue. What we should be concerned about is fat, not weight.

Being overweight is merely weighing more than the standardized height/weight tables that tell you what you should weigh. Being obese refers to the percentage of fat that is on your body. There is a big difference. For example, you can have two men who are 6'2" tall and weigh 235 pounds. One man plays halfback for the Los Angeles Rams and the other is a less active male citizen. According to the height/weight charts, both are overweight since they shouldn't exceed 198 pounds. However, when you ask both men to take off their shirts, there is an obvious difference between the two. The professional football player has minimal body fat and a high distribution of lean body tissue. He looks very good. The other gentleman carries a large amount of fat and has very little lean body tissue. He doesn't look so good. Yet according to the charts, both are in the same "shape."

Many people panic at the sight of an unwanted pound. Yet in their fight to ward off pounds, they've ignored what happens to their bodies. They're adept at losing weight but not fat. In other words, they may lose lean body tissue yet gain body fat.

The key, you see, is lean body tissue; the bone, organ, and muscle tissue of your body. While you can't do much about your bones and organs, you can control the amount of muscle tissue you have. A person in good physical condition will have a high distribution of lean body tissue and a low distribution of fat. A person who is unfit will have a reverse distribution.

Now that puts a different twist in the whole weight-loss issue. For you see, you need to lose fat, not weight. Unfortunately, you cannot assume that losing weight automatically means that you're losing fat. What you can assume, however, is that when you lose weight through dieting you will lose both fat and lean body tissue. Hence, you become a scaled down version of the original model: 30 pounds lighter but still plagued with sagging muscles, a protruding stomach, flabby thighs, and a lack of energy.

Drs. Bill Zuti and Lawrence Golding conducted a study at Kent State University that illustrates this point. The research team set out to compare the effects of several different methods of weight reduction on body weight, body composition, and selected blood measurements. The 25 women participating in the study were all between the ages of 25 and 40, and were 20 to 40 pounds overfat. Three groups were formed: 1) eight women were put on a diet to reduce their caloric intake by 500 calories per day, but they held their physical activity constant; 2) nine continued to eat as usual, but increased their physical activity to burn off 500 extra calories a day; and 3) eight reduced caloric intake by 250 calories a day and increased their physical activity to burn off 250 calories a day. Before and after the 16-week period, the subjects were tested for body weight, body density, skinfold and girth measurements, and selected blood fats.

The results indicated that there were no significant differences between the groups in the amount of weight lost. In all three groups the average individual loss was 11.4 pounds. Thus, the study indicated that all of the methods were extremely effective in controlling weight. However, the significant finding of the study was that there was a difference between the groups with regard to body composition. Those in the exercise group and in the combination exercise/diet group had undergone significant changes in body density. The dieting group lost both body fat and muscle tissue; the exercise group lost more body fat and no muscle tissue. The report concluded that the use of exercise in a weight reduction program is far superior to dieting alone in its effect on body composition.

When people lose weight by dieting they often remain flabby. But if you exercise while you diet or use exercise as the means for losing weight, your muscles will be much firmer. Therefore, you will look and feel better after losing weight through exercise than you will after just dieting.

The reason for this lies in an understanding of the fat-loss principle. Basically, there is one way to lose fat: establish a caloric deficit. That simply means that you burn off more calories than you take in. If the calories in the foods we eat are not used, they are stored as fat To lose the extra poundage, you have two choices: decrease the amount of food you eat, or increase the amount of calories you use.

The Woes of Dieting

The most obvious and most often used method to lose extra poundage is to diet. It seems to make sense. "If I'm 500 calories over my limit, the best way to lose weight is to cut 500 calories out of my daily diet. Cut back on portions, no desserts, and no snacks." The only problem is that 95 percent of those people who lost weight through dieting gain it right back. The reasons why follow.

First, dieting is "unnatural." It works against the body's own wants and needs. You are a creature that is made to eat. Eventually your body will cry for more food and you will respond. Hence, the diet is disregarded. In addition to being unnatural, dieting is loaded with psychological stumbling blocks. Eating has been linked to emotional needs that are as compelling as actual hunger. We eat when we're nervous. We eat when we're bored. We reward ourselves with food when we are happy. We soothe ourselves with a big meal when we are sad. As children, we were good little boys or girls if we cleaned up our plates. We could have a candy bar if we behaved. Our Little League coaches even took us to the ice cream stand if we won the ball game. So the very act of dieting is psychologically interpreted as punishment, and no one likes to be punished for very long.

In addition to all that, dieting simply goes against everything our culture demands from us. In our society, food is plentiful. It's everywhere. It's also big business. "You're the one," because "you deserve a break today," so why not have a hamburger, a malted shake, or french fries? Radio, TV, magazine advertisements, and giant billboards all proclaim food as being fun and readily available right around the corner. Food advertisers know how to appeal to our cravings in a way that only the strongest can resist.

There's one other reason I'm down on diets, and that is that dieting robs you of energy. You see, we have been so conditioned about weight loss through dieting that we have forgotten the purpose of food. Simply stated, we *need* food to live, and we need a balanced, adequate amount of food each day in order to have the energy to carry out our daily activities. When a person who normally consumes 2,500 calories decides to starve off 250 of those calories each day, he is simply depriving himself of the fuel he needs to work and play. There is a good deal of indirect evidence to support this. If you'd take a look at the caloric requirement tables issued by the World Health Organization of the United Nations, you would see that they suggest 2,400 calories for a "sedentary" man while 4,500 calories are recommended for a "very active" man. Hard-working laborers, military personnel, and athletes require 6,000 or more calories per day, according to this organization. In other words, more "fuel" is needed for people who require a lot of energy. It has been estimated that Olympic-class swimmers must take in approximately 6,000 to 8,000 calories while on their grueling training. They require a great deal of energy, and without the extra fuel they would not be able to work as hard.

The implications are obvious. Dieting depletes our fuel supply, hence creating an energy shortage. That shortage is experienced far too often by dieters and the result is a drastic reduction in activity and the drive to conserve fuel. It's like starting off in third gear. The engine barely has enough energy to get you going. I'm afraid that's the way many dieters feel.

Finally, dieting does not help your body to look fit. So you're still depressed, despondent, dejected, and de-energized. You may temporarily drop 15 or 20 pounds, but your body will still have that "soft" look. You may still have a bit of a midriff bulge or flabby thighs. That's because dieting does not discriminate. It takes off pounds whether they be muscle or fat. I'm sure you've heard some say, "I lose weight, but I lose it in all the wrong places." For women, this usually means the diet unloaded 4 pounds *and* two inches from her bust. For men, the protruding stomach may stay while the biceps dwindle, adding to that pear-shaped, somewhat limpid look. The Golding-Zuti study I mentioned earlier illustrated just this point.

With all this going against you, why diet? I can see no sound reason to subject yourself to such energy-draining abuse, especially since there is an alternative; one that not only works directly to increase your energy, but is fun too! Instead of thinking negatively (don't eat this, none of that), think positively (add ten minutes here, treat yourself to an extra game of tennis). The key to slimming for energy is a regular program of aerobic activity.

Assessing Your Condition

Before beginning your program, you need to assess your conditions. Are you indeed obese? There are a number of ways to find out, but remember, we are concerned with body fat, not body weight. Physiologists measure this in terms of percentages. As I mentioned before, ideally, a woman should have about 19 percent fat on her body, while a man should have 15 percent. If you exceed those percentages, you are accumulating too much fat. If a man exceeds 25 percent and a woman 29 percent, they enter the range of obesity, and a world of very little energy.

Measuring Skinfold Thickness

The National Center of Health Statistics in Washington points out that "skin folds permit a closer estimate of body fat than do the tables of relative weight. Skin folds are becoming established as the easiest and most direct measure of body fat available in the doctor's office, the clinic, or in a large-scale population survey."

In most people under the age of 50, at least half of the body fat is stored directly underneath the skin. By measuring the thickness of the fold produced when the skin and tissue just under it are firmly grasped, it is possible to get a good idea of how much fat is present. Some of the most common locations at which this measurement is taken include the upper arm at the triceps (back of upper arm), the subscapular region (middle of the back at the shoulder blades), the waistline, the biceps (front of upper arm), and the ilium (waistline right above the hipbone).

The Pinch Test

Calipers are precise and scientific, but you're not conducting a research survey. You don't need to caliper to measure your own skinfold to determine whether or not you are fat. Simply do the pinch test.

Gently pinch the skin at the triceps of one upper arm (at the back), midway between the shoulder and elbow (with the thumb and forefinger of the other hand). Ideally, the skinfold should be between 1/4 and 1/2 of an inch. If you can grasp more than 1 inch, you can probably conclude you are sliding into the obese range.

The Chest/Waist Test

Here's another way to tell if you're too fat. Stand with your shoulders pulled back and *maximum* chest expansion. Measure the circumference of your chest just below the armpits. Be certain your tape measure is flat and level. Then measure your waist (at the navel), with your stomach in a relaxed position—not sucked in or forced out. For men, the chest should be five inches greater in circumference than the waist; for women, the difference should be ten inches. If your chest/waist difference is *less* than the five or ten inch criteria, you may conclude that you are carrying too much fat.

Weight Gain Test

A third test is to simply recall what you weighed when you were 18 if you are a woman, or 21 if you are a man. If memory fails, you can dig out old medical records. You can assume that each pound gained since that time represents an accumulation of fat.

Note: If you were obese at 18 or 21 and have lost weight, this test doesn't apply. Furthermore, if you have gained a lot of weight because you have been on a weight-training program, the test will also be invalid.

The Mirror Test

The quickest, easiest way to find out if you are too fat is to get undressed and stand in front of a full-length mirror. Do you like what you see? Have your body contours changed? If you look fat, you can reasonably conclude that you *are* fat. If you sag where you don't want to sag, if your abdomen protrudes, you may be moving into the obese range or are already there.

Ask yourself the following questions.

1. Does your stomach protrude?
2. Are your hips too big?
3. Do you have saddlebags on the tops of your thighs?
4. Do your breast or chest muscles sag?
5. Do you have handlebars above your hips?
6. Do the back of your arms seem flabby?
7. Do your legs seem to have the cottage cheese look?
8. Are your ankles too big?

If the answer is yes to any of these questions, you are probably carrying too much fat. Just be careful that you aren't too hard on yourself when you do the mirror test. Younger women especially are apt to want to measure up to a fashion model's ideal figure which, unless you are built along lean, long ectomorphic lines, is probably not possible nor even desirable.

The Jiggle Test

If the mirror test doesn't tell you too much, you might try running in place while standing in front of the mirror without your clothes on. If parts of your body jiggle and they're not supposed to, you can conclude that what you see jiggling is fat, and should be lost. If you still can't figure it out, look at your thighs, abdomen, and jowls or chin.

By now you should have a pretty good idea of whether or not you are carrying around too much fat to have the energy you would like to have. The problem, of course, is how to remove that fat so that you can really *live* rather than just exist. Since my plan is based on *using* calories rather than restricting calories, activity is the foundation for getting rid of that energy-robbing fat. I'd like to tell you that it's easy, and that it's effortless. That's what all the advertisements say about the gadgets and pills that promise to melt away your fat. I have to be more realistic, though, and tell you that while using activity to reduce fat is easier than dieting, it still takes a degree of self-discipline and determination.

The Inches-Off, No-Diet Plan

Calories are quite familiar to people concerned about their weight. Most know which foods are low in calories and which foods have high caloric content. Many have memorized the exact caloric values of a wide variety of foods. In other words, the calorie has been thought of mainly as something one eats, but hardly ever as a unit of energy, as fuel to thrive on.

Although many people count the number of calories they eat each day, the idea of counting the number of calories they burn is relatively new. My entire fat-loss principle is predicated on burning more calories than you eat. The program depends on getting an initial read on your individual calorie intake and calorie outgo. While it would be ludicrous to claim that keeping track of the calories that one burns is fun, it is certainly no more difficult than the traditional routine of counting the number of calories consumed. It's just different.

Everything You Need to Know about Calories

The calories your body requires just to keep going may be quite a few more or less than what some other person's body needs to keep from grinding to a halt. One reason for this difference is your individual basal metabolic rate. Roughly defined, the basal metabolic rate is the rate of energy turnover—measured while the person is sleeping or at rest—necessary to sustain all of the body's vital processes. This basal metabolic rate, in turn, depends upon several factors. One of the most important factors is your body size. Most people who weigh from 100 to 120 pounds burn about 50 to 60 calories per hour while at rest. People who weigh from 150 to 170 pounds usually burn 65 to 80 calories per hour while at rest.

In the same way, one individual can burn a significantly different number of calories during activity than another person burns. Variations depend upon age, level of fitness, sex, skill, nutrition, environmental conditions and, very importantly, body size. For instance, during an hour of gardening, a 200-pounder will burn approximately 430 calories, while a person weighing 100 pounds will burn only about 285 calories—much the same way that a large automobile uses more gas than a little economy model does to go the same distance.

How to Determine Your Caloric Outgo and Intake

The six Activity Tables in Appendix A entitled "The Fat-Loss Calorie Counter" take into account these individual differences. Start by looking at the column headed by the number of pounds you weigh. In that particular column are listed the number of calories you burn while participating in the various activities listed at the left side of the table. You can then use Appendix B, the Calorie Content of Food, to assess the number of calories you consume in your daily meals and snacks. By comparing the two figures, you'll get an idea of just how many net calories your body is exchanging and, perhaps, keeping as glycogen, or fat.

A local schoolteacher I know is a good example of this (See Table 13-1.) In the warmer months, Ed is physically active on a regular basis. He does some running and cycling. He's more apt to walk rather than use his car. He plays tennis and enjoys working in his garden. Consequently, he has little trouble with excess fat. His eating habits don't change. In fact, it's not unusual for Ed to eat more during the summer than the winter. Yet the amount of calories he eats are balanced with the amount of calories he uses.

When winter rolls around, Ed becomes somewhat less active; nothing drastic. His bicycle stays in the garage. He finds the Michigan winter weather a bit too severe for running or walking outdoors. Of course, there's no garden work. He enjoys playing in a basketball league, but that's only once a week. Even though his eating habits remain the same, he always puts on a few unwanted pounds during the winter. That's because his caloric output has declined. He is not using as many calories as he does during the summer and he ends up with a surplus at the end of each day, only about 200 extra, in fact. But that's about two pounds of fat gained each month. A five-month winter could mean ten extra pounds for Ed.

To estimate your calorie expenditure, check Appendix A on page 206 to find out the number of calories you would burn if you slept 24 hours. This would be your basal caloric need. Add to this basal caloric need the following percentages, depending upon your personal lifestyle.

1. Add 20 percent to the basal caloric need for bed patients or people confined to wheelchairs.

2. Add 30 percent for individuals who have only limited physical exercise. These would include ambulatory hospital patients and people convalescing from serious illness.

3. Add 40 percent for individuals who are not convalescing, but are doing very little work. Most housewives who engage in many social activities and have someone to do their housework would fall into this category. Students and secretaries who do not engage in regular exercise would also fall into this category; most office workers who do not engage in physical exercise on a regular basis would be included here. (Going once or twice a week does *not* qualify a person to move to a higher category.) The majority of people are in this particular range. If you are not on a regular exercise program place yourself in this category.

4. Add 50 percent for individuals who work steadily as cooks, domestics, and operators of various machines. Also in this group are students doing additional lab or library work at school, provided they stand and walk at least two hours daily. A housewife who does her housework and has pre-school children to care for is in this group.

5. Add 60 percent for most manual laborers—farmers and roofers—as well as for students who engage regularly in physical education classes or intramural sports activities. Also included are students who dance four or five times a week, provided that these students also walk or stand for two hours a day.

6. Add 70 percent for those who regularly engage in heavy work—construction workers and miners—and students who participate regularly in physical education classes, as well as intramural and interschool sports of a moderate nature (e.g., baseball).

7. Add 80 to 100 percent for those students who play and participate in vigorous intercollegiate or interschool sports, such as football, basketball, wrestling, track, field, or cross-country.

Table 13-1. Ed's Daily Caloric Exchange

ED'S DAILY INTAKE

BREAKFAST	CALORIES
1 bowl cereal with milk and sugar	250
1/2 grapefruit	50
2 pieces of toast with butter and jam	280
2 cups of coffee with cream and sugar	96

MID-MORNING SNACK	
donut	150
2 cups of coffee with cream and sugar	96

LUNCH	
2 sandwiches (cheese, tuna, etc.)	560
apple	75
2 cookies	65

AFTER SCHOOL	
1 cola	150
chips or peanuts	100

SUPPER	
Salad with dressing	150
meat	200
rice or potato	100
glass of milk	250
dessert	200

LATE NIGHT SNACK	
2 beers	300
nuts	50
TOTAL	3,122

ED'S DAILY OUTPUT

ACTIVITY	CALORIES
Driving car	100
Eating	95
Resting	320
Sitting/reading	380
Sleeping	525
Standing	105
Telephone	95
Typing	125
Washing dishes	140
Writing	95
Personal toilet	215
Calisthenics	292
Basketball	395
TOTAL	2,882

ADDITIONAL ACTIVITY IN SUMMER

Cycling to school	493
Tennis	225
TOTAL	718

To estimate your calories, simply consider how many pounds you seem to struggle with each year. Is it 5, 10, 15, or more pounds? Once you have established the number of pounds you gain, you can quickly estimate the number of calories you are out of balance. for every pound you gain yearly, you are out of caloric balance by 10 calories a day. Thus, if you have a 5-pound weight gain over a year's time, you are out of caloric balance by 50 calories a day. A 10-pound annual weight gain means a 100 calories-a-day imbalance.

Simply add this to the figure you received on the caloric outgo. For example, if you find out that you were burning off 2,200 calories a day as you work and play your way through the day and you are struggling with 10 pounds a year, you would be eating about 2,300 calories a day.

Now that you know how many calories you normally consume and how many calories you typically expend, life can be a lot more fun. In this energy-conscious age, the horrible task of counting calories can become one of the supreme pleasures in life—you can burn up all of the energy you want to, and it won't cost you a dime. Rather, you'll keep finding more and more energy.

A few examples are in order here. Let's assume that you're out of caloric balance by 100 calories a day. You go through the activity calorie counter (Appendix A) until you come to walking. Select the number of minutes it takes for you at your weight to burn 100 calories worth of activity. For example, if your present weight is 155 pounds, a half-hour stroll at 2 1/2 MPH—a nice leisurely pace, neither very slow nor very fast—will burn off approximately 100 to 125 calories per day and restore your caloric balance.

Of course, you want to lose fat, not just stay as you are. So, select a second activity. The best activities are those that are listed under aerobic exercise. A half-hour of target heart rate exercise usually burns about 300 calories. If you could manage a daily session, you would lose fat at the rate of almost three pounds a month.

You can supplement these activities with some other kinds of activities. Anything that burns extra calories is going to help you lose weight and fat. So the word "activity" as used here refers to anything that lets you move your muscles. It most definitely need not be "exercise" in the traditional sense of the word.

Housework—mopping, scrubbing floors, vacuuming, dusting—is an activity, and a pretty good one for burning off calories, as is lawn work, washing the car, painting the garage, chopping wood, or climbing stairs. However, with the exception of housework (which never ends, as everybody knows only too well), you couldn't very well plan a whole program based only on these other activities. Instead, it's best to regard these occasional muscle-movers as bonus activities. Their real value is supplementary. Do them as often as you can to boost your total weekly calorie expenditure.

In this program, the most rewarding activities are vigorous and involve the use of the whole body's muscles. Free-form modern dance, cycling, swimming, cross-country skiing, jogging, aerobics, running in place, walking, gymnastics, tennis, handball, volleyball, and many other sports are excellent.

Stationary exercises and calisthenics (the kind that have you reaching, bending, stretching, pulling, and kicking) are less valuable because most of them involve the use of smaller muscle groups. However, you can get good results from a routine of several kinds of stationary exercises if you put them together in such a way that the whole body gets a workout.

Strategies for Fat Fighting

14

It's quite likely that you wouldn't be reading this book if there wasn't an energy crisis within your body's economy. And, as you probably have gathered, the reason for this energy problem is that you've slipped into a lifestyle that uses energy faster than you can supply it. Your body is on the loser's end of a trade deficit—you're importing too much of the wrong kind of energy and exporting too little of the right kind of energy. Your body's energy crisis can only be cured by increasing exports so that you can once again be industrious, productive, and even have a bit of disposable energy so that you can participate in the extras of life that once were beyond your grasp.

If you've decided that you want to adopt a more active pattern of living, the best way to guarantee that you in fact do make the necessary changes is to make it official. Announce your intentions to your spouse or other trusted acquaintances. And don't stop there. Take steps toward building an environment for yourself that will encourage you to stick with your fat-fighting, energy-building approach to life.

Fat-Fighting Strategies

Here are some fat-fighting strategies that will make a difference over the long haul.

Exercise with a Friend...Maybe

We are all social beings, and enjoy doing things together. As you embark on a program of exercise and activity, try to get a friend to do it with you. When you go it alone, it's easy to skip a day or two. But if your friend is counting on you, it's harder to say no.

Exercising with a friend can be stimulating—for some people. My wife Beth picks up energy by being with people—a real extrovert. I'm different. I like to be alone. I seem to regroup by giving myself some quiet time. My run gives me the perfect opportunity. It's quiet time, and the solitude energizes my batteries. Find what works best for you.

Exercise at the Same Time Each Day

In addition to being social creatures, we are creatures of habit. Take a look at the things that really count in your daily life. They occur at roughly the same time each day. By choosing a particular time of day to do your exercise, it becomes part of your routine and thus more difficult to forget. It's important to choose a time of day when you are "up." If you are a morning person, try to exercise in the morning. If it takes you quite a while to get started in the morning, do your exercise before supper just after you get home from work. Soon, you will look forward to the time that you have set aside to do your body and mind a great favor.

Pick an Activity You Enjoy

You hate running? Then don't run! You have always enjoyed riding your bike? Then make that your basic activity for losing fat. Too many times we think of exercise as a form of punishment. We rigidly put ourselves through the paces, much like a drill instructor at boot camp. No wonder so many people say, "I just don't like to exercise!" Choosing something you like to do will help you to stick with it longer and see results quicker. Activities you hate become boring. Boring activities produce fatigue or a low level of energy.

Dress the Part for Activity

This may seem like an insignificant bit of advice, but you'd be surprised what it does for your mind to go through the procedure of changing into a T-shirt, shorts, sweat pants, or athletic shoes. There's a little bit of fantasy in each of us, and sometimes when I lace up my running shoes, I'm mystically transported to the starting line of the prestigious Boston Marathon as one of the leading contenders for the individual title. I know that sounds far out, but I've found that it works for more runners than just myself. Have your special "outfit" for whatever activity you choose.

Think the Part

Get psyched up! If you go out for a jog or a walk thinking negatively, there's no way you will enjoy it. Picture your heart, lungs, and arteries working together efficiently to provide your body with energy-giving oxygen. Get fired up about the fact that you are part of a unique group of individuals who care enough to do something for their bodies. Take pride in the fact that you are *doing* rather than sitting.

Do it to Music

If the activity you choose is something that's done indoors, by all means, put on your Walkman or turn on the radio. Choose music that you enjoy, but also music that is up to tempo. It's a great motivator. Once, when running late at night in the fieldhouse of a local college, one of the students put a record on the P.A. system. It was like a tonic. The music came loudly over the speakers and you could feel the beat all through the fieldhouse. I noticed my pace picked up without even thinking about it, and I kept that pace much longer than I normally would have.

Add Active People to Your List of Friends

Once you start exercising regularly, you will soon discover that you're not the only one doing it. You'll meet people in the park where you walk, at the health club where you lift weights, or at the gymnasium where you play basketball. As you make acquaintances with these people, you will find that physical activity becomes a common denominator for friendship. You will soon find that you enjoy meeting and being with these people to share advice and encouragement as you pursue the active life.

Avoid Sitting Before and After Supper

Perhaps the most common eating routine in America is this: Set down the lunch box, open the refrigerator, grab a snack, sit down in front of the TV, eat supper, retire to the easy chair in front of the TV, read the paper, watch the news, have another snack, and go to bed. These poor eating habits are conducive to gaining fat and certainly aren't very energetic. To break that routine, try to stay on your feet before and after supper. Spend the time working on a project around the house or with a hobby. Or spend it with your family. When you watch the news, try doing some light calisthenics or stretching exercises on the floor of the living room as you watch.

Avoid Overdoing It

I had a friend who bought fertilizer for his lawn one spring. The directions told him to spread it at a certain rate, which he did. Then he reasoned that going back over his lawn again would give it a double dose and therefore do that much better. So, he went back over his lawn again with the fertilizer. Within a week, the grass was brown. It sounds crazy, yet some people do this with exercise. In your effort to return to an energetic life, remember that it takes time. For every year that you have been inactive, you should plan on at least a month to get back into a better physical condition. So if you have been sedentary for ten years, it will take ten months for you to reach a level of fitness with which you can be happy. Take your time and have patience.

Look at "Before" Pictures

As you begin to make progress toward a slimmer and more energetic you, get some old photographs out and take a look at what you once looked like. Not only will you have trouble believing that you were ever that fat, you will also resolve to never get that way again. Hence, you will keep up with your program.

Tell People about Your New Way of Life

As you share your success with others, you will strengthen your own resolve in continuing to lead an active life. You may even find that some people look to you for advice. You may even become the resident expert on fitness in your neighborhood. There's nothing wrong with that. In fact, it's just one of the many rewards for doing something positive to take care of your body.

Chart Your Progress

If you walk, jog, run, or cycle, use a map to keep track of the distance you've covered. It's kind of fun to be able to tell others that you ran to Hawaii and back. If your activity can't be measured in miles, measure it in minutes. Within a short time, you'll be able to say something like, "I played tennis for 78 days!"

Use Your Legs Rather Than a Car

This will not only improve your own energy, it will help to ease the nation's energy crisis. Set a minimum limit. Never use the car for distances less than one mile, two miles, or even three miles.

Obviously, this list is not exhaustive. It primarily emphasizes activity. Supplement it with your own ideas. For example, one friend of mine insists upon eating a filling, well-balanced meal before going grocery shipping. He has discovered that by doing this he is less likely to impulsively pluck packages of scrumptious-looking food off the shelves. Then, back home when his defenses are down and he feels like snacking, nothing is available but nuts, apples, and other nutritious food.

If you stick with the program, as the weeks go by you'll notice definite progress. If you're like many fat-fighters I know, you'll enjoy keeping track of the disappearing pockets of fat. The scales are only one way of doing this. The pinch, jiggle, mirror, and other tests described in Chapter 13 are better techniques. Also, by listening to your body, you will soon "feel" definite improvements after only a few weeks of activity. Your breathing will come easier. Your heart rate may slow down by several beats a minute. Your energy level will reach a new high.

As you achieve these improvements, celebrate. Have a picnic in the park, take the family to the beach, or go skiing with a friend. Enjoy doing something that you've always wanted to do but never found the time for. Even running an extra mile can qualify as a celebration.

Realize, however, that there will be no cause for celebration unless you put your strategies for fat-fighting into action. To help you get started, you may want to use the three phase plan at the end of this section, which is based on the principles just described.

This three phase plan is designed around choosing two activities that you will enjoy doing on a regular basis. The first activity is to get you back into caloric balance (make calorie output equal intake). I call this your caloric balancer. The second activity is to establish a deficit so that weight is actually lost rather than maintained—your fat-burner activity.

A Three-Phase Plan for Slimming

No one likes to admit being too fat. We prefer to use descriptions like "pleasantly plump," "a little heavy," or "big boned." The tests at the end of Chapter 13 will help you come up with an honest evaluation of whether or not you are too fat. I suggest that you go through each test and answer every question. If the majority of the tests indicate that you are carrying too much fat, I would suggest that you begin with Phase One. If, however, you are generally pleased with the way you look, but sense the need to drop a few pounds, it might be better for you to begin at Phase Two. Phase Three is for people who already have their weight under control, and want to maintain that level of slim living.

Phase One: The Caloric Balancer Program

Phase One is your introduction to a better-looking body. This program of brisk walking will get your body into shape for the time when you actually engage in target heart rate exercise. Walking is also beneficial to your cardiovascular system. It's mild enough for almost everyone to enjoy. You will not *lose* a great deal of weight in Phase One. Instead, you will quit gaining weight as you burn off those extra calories.

Phase One: Walking Program (6-7 Times per Week)

STEPS*	DURATION OF EXERCISE (MINUTES)
1	15-17
2	18-20
3	21-23
4	24-26
5	27-29
6	30-33
7	34-37
8	38-41
9	42-44
10	45-50

*Spend a *minimum* of one week at each step in the phase.

Bonus Activities

In addition to your caloric balancer program, Phase One will introduce you to the concept of "building activity into your life." That simply means that you will try to find ways to use your body to do things instead of finding ways to avoid using it. The 10 to 12 extra calories you might use doing things the "hard way" will add up and help you to maintain your weight. Select one of the following suggestions and program it into your life while you are working on Phase One.

1. Don't use the escalator or elevator if there are stairs.
2. Don't drive if you can get there by bicycle or foot.
3. When you drive, park at the far end of the parking lot so that you have to walk a little bit more to get to your destination.
4. Don't use an electric mixer, blender, or can opener if you can do the job by hand.
5. Don't use a power saw if a hand saw will do the job.
6. Don't use a dryer if you have a clothes line out in the yard, to help you bend and stretch.
7. While you watch television, get up and walk in place or bend and stretch during each commercial and station break.

In addition to selecting one of those activities, try to follow these five suggestions in all that you do:

1. Never lie down when you can sit up.
2. Never sit when you can stand. The caloric difference per hour is 10 calories, which is enough to have a discernable effect over the months.
3. Get into the habit of "pacing"; instead of dropping into a chair to mull over a problem, get up and move around.
4. As a general rule, never sit for more than an hour and a half without standing, stretching, and walking for five minutes or so.
5. Run in place whenever you can, even if it is only for 30 seconds or so. Time spent waiting is a natural for this.

Phase Two: The Fat-Burner Program

This phase combines walking, a target heart rate activity, and bonus activities that will help you to lose fat. The walking will help you to maintain a balance in your caloric output/input. Though you may have already lost some pounds through this activity, the real weight loss will come with your second activity—the fat burner.

You have several options for your target heart rate activity. You can run, swim, cross-country ski, aerobic dance, run in place, jump rope, and of course, continue walking. As you do the fat-burner exercise, you should be pushing your heart rate up to about 60 percent of your maximum heart rate. (See Chapter 9 for a more detailed description of your target heart rate.)

Phase Two: Fat-Burner Program (4 Times per Week)

Steps*	Caloric Balance or Walking (Minutes)	Target Heart Rate Activity (Minutes)
1	30	10
2	27	13
3	25	15
4	22	18
5	20	20
6	17	23
7	15	25
8	15	28

*Spend a *minimum* of two weeks at each step in this phase.

Bonus Activities

In Phase One you selected one bonus activity to work on while you were going through that phase. For Phase Two, select an additional activity and work on it while you are going through each step of this phase.

Phase Three: The Super Slimming Program

By the time you reach Phase Three, you will be a veteran, one of those exercisers you used to admire. The first step of Phase Three is the minimum goal of most people who are interested in reducing their body fat, because at this step you're getting 30 minutes of target heart rate exercise. This is a very realistic goal that almost anyone can reach. Stick to it and you will not only wipe out your problem, you will find yourself in fine physical condition. You will forget that energy was ever a problem.

At this level the caloric balancer part of your program (walking) can be done at any time. Just make sure you do it. Do it on your way to work, or during your lunch break. The amount of time spent at each step is up to you. You may be satisfied with 30 minutes of heart rate activity four times a week. Your weight loss may be gradual and sustained, and that amount of time may just fit perfectly into your daily schedule. On the other hand, you may want to progress slowly through each step, enjoying continued weight loss and improved fitness. As a rule, spend at least two weeks at each step. Don't be too eager. The important thing is to stick to the program on a regular basis.

Phase Three: Super Slimming Program (4 Times per Week)

Steps*	Caloric Balance or Walking (Minutes	Target Heart Rate Activity (Minutes)
1	15	30
2	15	33
3	15	35
4	15	38
5	15	40
6	15	43

*Spend a *minimum* of two weeks at each step in this phase.

Bonus Activities

Go back to the bonus activities listed in Phase One and try to include as many of them as possible in your daily routine. Your goal is to become an active person. That is, a person who finds pleasure in using his/her body to do things. Here's an encouraging thought: When you reach Phase Three of the eating plan and the slimming plan, fatness will no longer be a problem for you.

▶▶ *Relating to Others* ▶▶▶

The High Cost of Lousy Relationships

15 ▶▶▶

Picture this: It's 7:30 a.m. in the townhouse of Jane and John. They have been married for six years and both have successful careers. John is a bit edgy about a contract he will be working on at the office. Jane is a bit nauseated; nothing serious, but she just doesn't feel real great. John got up a little earlier than usual and made breakfast. Jane didn't feel like eating. John was hurt and said something that upset Jane. Then Jane said something back to John and before long, sharp words were being exchanged. Soon, it was icy quiet. At 7:50 a.m. they kissed, almost on signal, grabbed their attache cases, got in separate cars, and went to their respective jobs.

Silly, right? Almost like a soap opera. But the story's not over. At the office, John arrives rushed and harried. He closes his door, then begins pacing back and forth. At first, he is angry. Soon, however, his anger turns to worry. Maybe he was a bit harsh, he thinks. He really loves Jane and just can't seem to concentrate with this conflict unresolved. When he calls Jane's store he's told she's busy with a client. Now John is suspicious. He thinks Jane is still ignoring him. That makes him worry more. He decides he'd better sort through his mail to get his mind off of his troubles with Jane. He opens a letter and reads it three times before he realizes he isn't reading it at all. He's thinking about Jane.

I think you get the idea. John has become almost totally immobilized with worry over what he perceives to be a break in his relationship. If we followed him around the rest of the day we would watch him spin his wheels,

153

expend a lot of energy, and get virtually nothing accomplished. Assuming that he gets things patched up at home later than night, the next day he will face two day's worth of work that probably needed to be finished yesterday. If I know John and Jane, it will only be a few days before they repeat their little argument.

You may think this little scenario I cooked up is a bit out of the ordinary. I wish it was. Unfortunately, it appears that far too many people are engaged in the types of relationships that prevent them from living a dynamic, energetic life. Just look around you. Marriage, often thought of as the ultimate relationship, is at best an "iffy" proposition. Of every 100 couples who marry, 50 of them will divorce. Over half of the remaining couples will experience such turmoil in their marriages that they would like to sever the relationship, but feel too trapped to do so. That means that roughly 20 to 25 percent of all marriages are based on sound, positive relationships.

Though divorce is the most dramatic example of a negative relationship, it isn't the only one. One of the trademarks of this generation is the decline of the traditional family unit. Relationships between parent and child are suffering. The number of teenage runaways increases each year. The lack of harmony between teachers and students in public high schools is frightening. The hostility among the students themselves is even more frightening. And to describe the relationship between employers and their employees, we often use terms like "contract," "bargaining," and "strikes." People are having a tough time getting along with each other.

As far as I'm concerned, there are two kinds of relationships: those that grow and develop and are alive, and those that are in a constant state of disrepair. Both are directly related to your energy level. The dynamic, positive relationship with another human being is just the ticket for an energetic life. It can be a source of inspiration and motivation. Even the most demanding days can be made more tolerable when you know you have support from someone who cares about you.

On the other hand, negative relationships produce a sense of turmoil that merely adds to the problems that you already have. When all of your energy is spent trying to shore up the breaks in a crumbling relationship, you have little energy left over to function as a normal member of society. Somehow, the bounce leaves your step, fatigue sets in earlier, and the inability to get things done becomes a real problem. You become immobilized. That is, because of your shaky relationship, your resolve to accomplish something has become weakened. That weakening may range from mild hesitancy or indecision to almost total inaction. Either way, you are not functioning at an optimum energy level.

This does not necessarily mean that you don't have any energy. Indeed, when you are forced to cope with a negative relationship, you often have a great deal of energy. If you will recall Dr. Hans Selye's explanation for how we handle stress, you will remember that during the alarm and resistance stage, tremendous amounts of adrenaline, and other hormones are secreted, peaking our energy supply to optimum levels. That is why, after an argument with another person, you are often hyped up. Your heart beats faster. Your blood pressure rises. You're really charged up. At the time, energy does not seem to be a problem.

What *is* a problem is where all that energy is being directed. Instead of being used to produce satisfying results, that surge of energy is being thrown into the fray. You're pacing, worrying, arguing, fuming, mulling, and sulking. When you finally get around to things that really matter, you're yawning. You've used up all that energy in the fight so that now you don't feel like typing up that report or playing catch with your kids.

Dr. James Lynch of the University of Maryland Medical School has stated that loneliness (even among the married), a lack of sound relationships, and high social mobility can cause a person to be hostile, angry, and frustrated, a deadly group of attitudes that are definitely not energy producing. That is why I call these types of relationships counterproductive. They produce just what you wish they wouldn't produce. Instead of harmony, support, acceptance, love, and satisfaction, counterproductive relationships produce worry, anxiety, stress, dissatisfaction, and turmoil. Furthermore, they take up so much of your time and energy that there is little of either left to devote to your job, hobbies, and other interests.

Unfortunately, things just don't stop with those feelings and reactions. And that's why interpersonal relationships are such an important area in discussing energy. As humans, we often allow one reaction to foster another one. Physiologists and psychologists like to describe such patterns as "syndromes." In this case, feelings of worry and stress created by counterproductive relationships lead us on the search for a quick fix. The executive who is unable to function at the office because of problems at home may turn to alcohol and/or tobacco to calm him down. He reasons it would be better to pour himself a drink to escape the immediate upheaval. Of course, the quick fix only masks the real reason for being upset, and puts off the eventual confrontation. It does not solve the problem.

One reason counterproductive relationships exist is because they are usually founded on improper motives. A genuine, positive relationship is a feeling of emotional bonding with another person in a positive way. It's a connection in which your heart and mind unite with that of another human being in such a way that both feel a sense of gratification. Although emotion is an important element, it is the communication—the sharing of those emotions—that nurtures and develops a relationship. A positive relationship involves both giving and sharing, with the other person's feelings in mind. If you would observe some of the relationships around you (or perhaps evaluate some of your own), you will find that there is often an imbalance between the giving and sharing. For some reason, the relationship is based more on circumstances, obligations, the need for approval, or personal gain. Whatever the cause, these relationships produce negative feelings and become counterproductive. Let's look at each of these more carefully.

Relationships Based on Circumstances

Stop and think of all the people you come in contact with throughout each week. In many cases, you develop relationships with those people. You may ride to work in a car pool. Your desk may be situated close to another employee in your office. You may rub shoulders with neighbors, salesmen, and repairmen. While these occasional contacts may not develop into full-fledged relationships, they often present situations that create stress and negative feelings.

For example, I have an associate who rides to work in a pool with four other people. The other day he said to me, "Charlie, I'm about to go back to driving my own car to work, even though it will cost more." When I asked why, he told me about one of the riders that was beginning to get on his nerves. "All he ever does is complain. Nothing suits him. The rest of us spend the entire trip trying to buoy his spirits or sympathizing with him. By the time I get to work I feel like I've already put in a few hours. I have lost a good bit of my energy."

It makes sense that other people can rob you of or give you energy. In his fine book, *The Art of Human Relationships,* psychologist Henry Clay Lingren notes that "whatever we are or what we have become...is influenced to the greatest extent by the thoughts, beliefs, and actions of people among whom we spend our lives." If a friend or an acquaintance is depressed, there is a tendency for you to pick up these feelings.

There is little that you can do about these types of relationships. You can't entirely avoid them. After all, you are a social animal. One of the responsibilities of living in a civilized society is having to relate to other people. Many times, that means striking up conversations or engaging in activities with people who rub you the wrong way. Since we normally like to avoid conflict, we often develop a grin-and-bear-it attitude. That is, even though we may be seething about having to relate to a particular individual inside, we act as if we enjoy his or her company.

Such playacting can seriously affect your energy level by creating stress. And the peculiar thing about this kind of stress is that it's often hard to pinpoint. You may really love your job, but find that one of the people you work with is very difficult to get along with. When you experience nervousness and anxiety in the morning as you get ready for work, you may mistakenly attribute it to your job, even though the problem may be that co-worker. The negative relationship has produced feelings that trigger the stress response, and eventually your job gets the blame for it.

These types of negative relationships cause people to lose control over their own immediate environment. We do all sorts of silly things to avoid having to deal with the relationship. I've known people who will wait until their neighbor goes indoors before they go outside to work in the garden simply because they don't want to have to struggle with a shaky relationship. Others decline invitations to entertainment because they are afraid "you-know-who" will also attend. Still others react by going overboard. They become back-slapping, apparently carefree sociables who go out of their way to display their affection toward the very people they wish to avoid, having learned such behavior prevents any real relationship from developing.

Whatever the reaction, it is usually not one that most people find satisfactory, and it creates a feeling of impotence. Instead of enjoying positive relationships with people of like mind and interests, the person trapped in a number of "circumstantial relationships" expends a lot of energy trying to avoid contact with others.

Relationships Based on Personal Gain

One of the curses of modern corporate society is called the "social ladder." No one likes to be called a "social climber," but the fact is that a great many attractive societal rewards are dealt on the basis of who your friends are. The young executive may not necessarily enjoy the company of his immediate superior, but he knows that if he wants to go anywhere in the company, he had better accept his social invitations, and better yet if he can garner an invitation from his superior's boss. Relationships on this level become vicious to the extent that they are used as weapons in a great upward-mobility war. In his book, *Executive Stress,* Harry Levinson notes the quickening pace at which young executives move up through the ranks of the company. He suggests there are more young people advancing more quickly to the top in shorter periods of time. One of the great causes of stress, says Levinson, is how the young executive "negotiates the social shoals." In his or her quest to achieve success, old friends are left behind and new ones are picked up that may enhance his or her rise in the company.

Relationships based on personal gain often have strings attached that can be a source of stress. The executive who forms relationships to enhance his career soon finds that he has little control over his social life. When the appropriate "friend" beckons, he must jump into action, often leaving behind favored activities and behaviors. Naturally, it is difficult to maintain such a relationship without a degree of resentment and bitterness. Since such relationships are crucial to success, they create a feeling of helplessness that can flavor one's entire outlook on life. Inevitably, the relationship produces such negative feelings that he becomes disillusioned, frustrated, and ineffective. All his energy is wrapped up in masking negative feelings while trying to use the relationship for personal gain.

In discussing this type of relationship, you may think I'm being too hard on executives. While executives may be most prone to this type of counterproductive relationship, they are not alone. At one time or another, practically everyone has been involved in a relationship of which the only purpose was personal gain. Students fresh out of college looking for jobs are told to make friends with the right kind of people. Politicians, seeking broad support from the electorate, make it their business to befriend virtually anyone with enough power to influence voters. Special-interest groups pay skilled lobbyists to mix and mingle with legislators. This is not to say all relationships developed in these areas are based on selfish reasons. Yet it is a simple fact that carefully selected friends can be used for personal gain. When the majority of your friends are merely pawns, even if used for noble purposes, you have put yourself into a stressful situation in which much of your energy is spent trying to keep those relationships afloat.

This isn't a problem reserved just for the big-league world of business, careers, or politics. It happens every day in good neighborhoods like yours and mine. The prevailing question in establishing relationships seems to be "What's in it for me?" The Joneses are more concerned about inviting the "right people" over, rather than people in whom they might truly be interested. Consequently, little value is obtained from such relationships. Instead of honest sharing and caring on a mutual basis, a great deal of energy is spent in posturing and posing to present a proper image. As far as I'm concerned, that's a lousy way to try to get along with people. It also explains the petty jealousies and needless backbiting that often accompanies these counterproductive relationships.

Relationships Based on Obligations

These relationships are closely related to relationships based on personal gain. In both cases, the relationship is artificial. Instead of a desire to communicate and share your thoughts, emotions, and beliefs with another human being, this type of relationship is formed because you feel you *have* to relate. Many times such relationships exist between in-laws: "Honey, why don't you take Dad to a ball game tonight?" Or sometimes you might feel obliged to form relationships because you belong to a service or fraternal organization: "Hey Harold, all the Guppies are expecting you to attend the next smoker!"

If the relationship based on personal gain causes anxiety and stress, relationships based on obligations can become even more immobilizing. That's because this type of relationship seems desperately inescapable. When you were making friends for some type of gain, you may have felt somewhat in control. At least you felt you would be rewarded with a promotion or some form of advancement. When your relationships are dictated to you by obligations, you feel like there's no way out.

Often, these types of relationships begin with a genuine need and desire for positive interaction and friendship. You may have joined a bowling team, neighborhood study group, bridge club, or service organization. The people you developed relationships with in these situations may be wonderful, caring people. Yet you soon discovered that your "free" time was being governed by the group's demands. Hence, every time you left the house to join them in an activity, you felt resentment and frustration. What should be a positive experience becomes depressingly negative. Instead of relaxation and recreation, it produces anxiety and stress. Such feelings, in turn, can create fatigue, depression, indecision, even immobilization.

Relationships Based on the Need for Approval

This is the one that often strikes the closest to home. Who doesn't want to win the approval of others? Very few people actually delight in being rejected. The rest of us will do practically anything for a good old pat on the back. Regardless of the size of your ego, you like to have it stroked now and then. In terms of counterproductive relationships, the problem comes when friendships are built on the need to be approved or accepted. When winning approval becomes the basis for developing a relationship, you become extremely vulnerable to the whim and fancy of everyone around you.

More serious than succumbing to the desires of others is the fact that such relationships are almost totally self-defeating. The beliefs, attitudes, hopes, and aspirations of everyone else become more important than your own. Soon you find yourself saying things you really don't mean just to avoid being disliked. Whenever someone disagrees with you, you become upset and depressed. Rather than carry on an intelligent conversation, you constantly shift your views and alter your position so that others won't disapprove. Eventually, you sacrifice your own self-concept and become totally dominated by others.

Unfortunately, many marriages struggle along with both parties caring more about seeking approval from each other rather than allowing each person to maintain a unique and independent identity. Wives feel guilty when their meals don't elicit raves from their husbands. Husbands become upset when wives don't show an interest in a recent success at the office, or vice versa. Success is judged according to what the other party thinks of you. The relationship becomes a tragicomic round of one-upmanship that has husband and wife doing all sorts of crazy things to win the approval of each other, and then experiencing guilt, worry, and anger when they think they have failed.

This is the case with Joe and Alice. Joe always felt that his wife deserved someone who could provide her with a higher standard of living than he could afford. So he works two jobs and even moonlights on Saturdays and Sundays to try to earn enough money to give her the lifestyle he always thought she wanted. Alice, in the meantime, felt bad because she never finished college. She felt inferior to Joe and noticed that he seemed most happy with people who had gone to college. So she enrolled as a part-time student at a community college and is struggling toward a degree.

Interestingly, Joe and Alice seldom see each other. As each strives to please the other, they are drifting farther and farther apart. Yet the sad part of this is that they genuinely love each other. What they need most is a relationship—some time to sit down and talk to each other. Then, they would find out that a lavish lifestyle won't make Alice happy and a college degree won't make Joe happy.

The effects of this type of relationship on your energy are quite clear. When all of your energy is directed toward winning approval from others, you have little left over for yourself. Poor Joe puts in 48 to 60 hours each week. He's a hard worker who really pushes himself. Yet whenever he manages to squeeze out a little spare time, he's too tired to do anything. And Alice can't even begin to consider enjoying a night out dancing or relaxing with a good book. She's too busy washing, ironing, taking care of the kids, and going to class. All of this because both have built their relationship on the need for approval from each other.

I know this chapter paints a pretty bleak picture of relationships. Lest you think I'm a pessimist, let me point out that, for many people, developing a relationship with another person is an exciting, invigorating experience. Personally, I have been blessed with many wonderful friends who are a constant source of inspiration and energy. Yet I'm afraid too many people are living defeated lives because of the negative relationships they are in. I am convinced they could lead more dynamic, energetic lives if these relationships were altered so that a genuine sense of sharing and an emotional bond could be formed.

All of us, at one time or another, have experienced some of the relationships described in this chapter. Dealing with them is difficult and often takes great courage. The next chapter will show you how you can transform a negative relationship into a positive one—move from a condition of wasted, misdirected energy to abundant energy. Now that you understand how relationships can be counterproductive, you can begin to nurture and cultivate the types of relationships that allow you *and* your friends to live dynamic lives.

Getting Energy through Giving and Getting Love

16 ▶▶

In the last chapter, I described ways in which relationships can produce a defeated life of anxiety, worry, frustration, and anger. I suppose one response to the threat of such relationships would be to avoid getting too close to anyone. Instead of risking a counterproductive relationship, you could insulate yourself from others and lead a safe, albeit lonely, life. Leading such a life, according to Dr. James Lynch, causes anger, hostility, and frustration. Indeed, this path seems popular for a great many people. Relationships are kept on a superficial level, with little chance of serious involvement. If you ask me, that's a lousy way to live.

There's hardly anything more stimulating than a lively conversation with a good friend. I'm sure you'll agree if you stop and think about it. Remember the last time you got together with a few people that you really liked and respected? You talked way on into the early morning hours, yet never really felt tired. Personally, I find such relationships extremely rewarding. But the relationship must go beyond conversation to be truly rewarding. It must embrace love and mutual caring.

Dr. George E. Vaillant, in his book *Adaptation to Life*, illustrates this point. Vaillant was involved in a long-term project that traced the personal growth and development of 268 American men over 40 years. These men were selected in the 1940's because they were supposedly the most promising undergraduates of a leading American university. They filled out detailed questionnaires about themselves at regular intervals. Then in 1969

Dr. Vaillant personally reinterviewed 94 of them in-depth. His comments on how these men influenced him illustrate a very important point about the way interpersonal relationships can make life energetic.

"I soon discovered that whether the men liked me or I liked them had far more to do with their lives than with mine. The men who had always found living easy made me feel warmly toward them, and led me to marvel at both my tact and my skill as an interviewer and at their good fortune to belong to such an enjoyable project. I left the office of one such man feeling ten feet tall; but he had had the same effect on others all of his life. In contrast, men who have spent their lives fearful of other people and had gone unloved in return often made me feel incompetent and clumsy. With them I felt like a heartless investigator, vivisecting them for science. During his interview one such man had confessed that he was afraid of dying and leaving nothing of worth to the world. Afterwards I, too, felt drained and depressed, as if I had done all of the work in the interview while he took much and gave nothing."

In short, a person's capacity and ability to love plays a key role on the impact he or she has on you. People who love, have fun, and care give you good feelings about yourself and your energy levels.

You already know a great deal about relationships and relating to others because you've been doing it ever since you were born. You have cultivated some relationships, rejected others, enjoyed some, and despised still others. All of your dealings with other human beings constitute relationships, but the question is, how do you make sure you have more positive relationships than negative ones? How can you add energy to your life by developing relationships that are mutually rewarding and meaningful? Like any form of self-directed change, it will take a little work. But I think you'll find that whatever you put into a positive relationship, you will receive double your money back.

The First Step

You'll never get along very well with others until you learn to enjoy your own company. Understanding yourself is essential before you can understand others and effectively relate to them. That may sound quite obvious to you, but it is an element that is missing from most relationships. The success or failure of a relationship depends almost entirely on your ability to love and respect yourself. Too many people use their relationships for everything but self-gratification. The relationships described in the last chapter are examples of this. Relationships became tools. They were used, not enjoyed—endured, not savored. Consequently, they produced feelings and emotions that fostered a paralyzing immobility.

I like the way Wayne Dyer defines self-love. He says it is "the ability and willingness to allow those that you care for to be what they choose for themselves, without any insistence that they satisfy you." That simply means that we shouldn't try to manipulate others when we form relationships. In order to love and accept people in this way, it is necessary that you be secure enough in yourself so that you no longer need others to be like you or need them to satisfy your own preconceptions of how they ought to act. When you reach this point, you will be able to love others and do things for them with no ulterior motives, but simply because you enjoy helping them.

I'll admit, that's hard. Being able to accept yourself—everything about you—is sometimes difficult. What about the physical side of you? Your body: Is it too tall, too short, too thin, too hairy? Is your hair too straight, are you teeth too crooked, your hips too flat? Now stop and think for a minute. Who's to say what's too hairy or too flat? Are you going to let fashion magazines dictate your self-concept? If so, things may get a little confusing. In the 1930's, models were flat-chested. In the 1950's, 36D was the "in" look. At any given moment, there is a look that's considered just right. Yet often, you must accept what Nature gave you. You can either fret and worry about it, or you can accept yourself and do the best with what you have. Once you can face yourself in a mirror and say, "It may not be perfect, but it's all I've got," you can begin to like yourself as a unique and wonderful human being. And when you arrive at that level of self-acceptance, you will find that it's easier to accept others. That's where sound, positive relationships begin.

Abraham Lincoln said something once that demonstrates this quality of self-acceptance: "If I were to read, much less to answer all the attacks made on me, this shop might as well be closed for any other business. I do the very best I know how—the very best I can; and I mean to keep doing so until the end. If the end brings me out all right, what is said against me won't amount to anything. If the end brings me out wrong, ten angels swearing I was right would make no difference."

So the first step to establishing positive relationships is to know, understand, and accept yourself. You'll discover that most of the things you want out of life are, in fact, attainable. You'll discover new energy as you pursue those goals simply because you are no longer bound by the paralyzing shackles of fear, self-doubt, and worry. You'll discover life is really fun because you are doing things that *you* want to do, not wasting your time and energy chasing other people's expectations. There's another added attraction to directing your own life: those who get the most approval are usually those who never seek it out.

Stand Up and Be Noticed

One of the major causes of those negative relationships described in the previous chapter was people refusing to assert themselves. I'm sure there have been many times when you wanted to disagree with someone or wanted to decline a social invitation. But you kept quiet because you didn't want to rock the boat. That type of behavior can lead to complete dominance of yourself by others. Perhaps your lack of energy is really due to the psychological halter that you're wearing, with everyone else leading you around and making your choices for you.

It's one thing to know and accept yourself. It's another thing to stand up for what you believe is right. Yet a healthy relationship is built on open and honest sharing. There's nothing wrong with you if your spouse doesn't agree with an idea you have. It's perfectly okay to tell your friends you'd just as soon not join them for a drink after work. Too many times we give away our freedom because we're more concerned about what others think than what we know is right for us.

I've known a lot of people who wanted to start jogging or walking but kept putting it off. They would tell me, "I feel so foolish, like everyone's staring at me." Amazing! Yet think of how many times you wanted to do something you felt was good or right, but other considerations kept you from doing it. You didn't want to be teased or kidded about it. You didn't want others to think that you were trying to be better than them.

Your relationships will become exciting and dynamic when you begin to feel free to assert yourself. People who really count will appreciate you more. Those who are more interested in dominating others will decide that they can no longer use you. That's okay. It may be necessary for some of those negative relationships to drop by the wayside. Chances are that you're wasting a lot of time and energy keeping them afloat. It's far better to have a few good relationships than a lot of lousy ones. Once you experience the freedom of knowing that your friends accept you for who and what you are, you'll never want to engage in another depressing, constricting relationship in which everyone counts but you.

Accepting Differences

Learning to accept and assert yourself will help you to establish relationships that give a tremendous amount of satisfaction. Learning to accept others, even if they hold different beliefs or values, will help even more. You will find that you're not limited to a certain group of people when it comes to choosing friends. Moreover, you will find it easier to relate on an informal basis with the various people that you come in contact with.

There are two possible reactions to individual differences. You can either resist and fear them or accept and use them. By now, you've learned that fear and resistance are low-energy terms. You can't possibly be on top of things if you are gripped with an attitude that restricts you. I've known people who choose friends much like they check out a used car. They're so concerned about the faults that they never really develop a relationship. They're too busy making sure that the other person fits into their own little value structure to see the potential of a good relationship.

On the other hand, there's a great deal of freedom that comes with letting go of the burdensome belief that everyone else should be just like you. When we give up this unrealistic assumption, we become free to allow others to be who they really are rather than enslave ourselves to the vain hope that they will be like us. When we truly believe it's all right for people to be different, we will stop developing relationships characterized by comparing, judging, disapproving, and manipulating.

Frankly, I find it supremely boring to constantly be around people who think and act just like me. Some of my closest friends are people who don't vote the same way I do, don't worship the same way I do, don't look the same way I look, and don't live the same way I live. Yet our relationships thrive on the insights and information that we can offer each other. I look forward to sharing with them. I am stimulated by our conversations. I am energized by our friendship.

Why people of different persuasions are stimulated and enjoy each other is an interesting phenomenon. After studying human relationships carefully, Eliot Chapple, an anthropologist, has concluded that we all have inherent rhythms in many human actions, including conversation. This means that people may be attracted to one another in conversation not just by the content of their talk but by the conversation rhythms. For example, if you are constantly interrupted by an acquaintance as you are speaking, your innate rhythms are dropped, regardless of how much you agree or disagree. Conversely, if you and a friend share mutual rhythms, the conversation will be stimulating, exciting, and energizing. I am sure, of course, that a conversation is stimulating to you if you find your counterpart to be intellectually exciting. But perhaps the excitement generated may be due to physiological rhythms.

Resolving Conflicts

Sometimes, even in the finest relationships, confrontation and conflict are necessary. In fact, they're essential. When there is a difference that needs to be hammered out, avoiding a confrontation is dishonest and builds a barrier. Eventually, this easy-way-out approach can destroy a relationship. You let the incident, however minor, build up inside of you. It eats away at your feelings, convincing you that there is real animosity between the two of you. Eventually, you let your anger show, words are exchanged, and the relationship can never be the same.

This happens a lot in marriages. People feel that an absence of conflict is an indication of a successful marriage. So they do everything imaginable to avoid conflict. Usually, they lie:

"Honey, is something bothering you?"

"No, of course not!"

When the conflict finally comes, a lot of repressed anger is released and another wedge is driven between them.

When conflicts arise, bring them out in the open and face them head-on. Usually, both parties involved will end up laughing at the insignificance of the whole thing. You'll be able to handle it in a shorter period of time and save yourself all the worry, frustration, and anger of the prolonged smoldering and the eventual explosion.

Another suggestion for dealing with conflicts in your relationships is to avoid getting angry. Anger is a handy tool for getting your own way. In a genuine relationship, you should be concerned less with getting your own way and more with assuring the survival and improvement of the relationship. Remind yourself that anger is a negative emotion, one that will produce undesirable results. As you feel yourself beginning to get angry, slow down. Try to jump out of your self and stand back from a distance to look at the situation. Or focus briefly on something totally unrelated to the conflict. These mental gymnastics help you to achieve a sense of objectivity and to put things back in proper perspective. If you can look out the window and see the sun and remind yourself that tomorrow it will rise again and the grass will still be green and the birds will still sing, you will return to the issue at hand calmer, more relaxed, and less insistent on being right.

The best advice I can give when it comes to resolving conflicts is to listen. Too many times people involved in conflict like to do a lot of talking. When they're not talking, instead of listening they are planning their next verbal barrage. By taking time to genuinely listen to the other person, you are first showing them respect, and second, obtaining some very useful information. Moreover, listening to someone as they share their side of the conflict can disarm any hostility that creeps in. If you would take the responsibility to be a good listener during your next conflict, you will probably discover that the conflict itself can be a positive experience, enabling your relationship to grow deeper.

When your turn comes to speak, avoid the usual accusatory, attacking statements or rhetorical questions that force the other person to go on the defensive. Any statement that begins with "You" will probably escalate the conflict.

"You never discipline the kids!"

"You always insist on getting your own way!" To avoid this, try a much more honest approach by stating directly how you feel. Share your emotions. Admit your insecurity or anger or whatever it is that is bothering you. Often, the incident is not what's important but the feelings that have resulted from the incident. Only after you repair those feelings can you begin to correct the cause of the conflict.

Handling conflicts positively is a great antidote to stress and anxiety. No doubt, you will continue to have conflicts in your relationships. As you learn to deal with them in a positive manner, those conflicts will take less energy to resolve. You will spend less time in petty bickering and more time enjoying each other's company.

Give It a Chance

Everything I've said about getting energy through giving love must be underscored with an important concept: there is no such thing as a quick fix to human relationships. I'm afraid one reason why so many relationships suffer is that people are too impatient. We are the "Now" Generation. If my friendships get me down, I'll get new friends. If my marriage isn't working, I'll scrap it and start over. If my kids and I don't get along, I'll give up— they'll be gone in a few years anyway.

Recognize that there are some problems which can be solved immediately, some which take time, and some that cannot be resolved. The key is to learn which are which and then learn to live with that concept.

Earn Your Neighbor's Love

The Bible admonishes us: "Thou shalt love thy neighbor as thyself." Significantly many other diverse religions and philosophies expound the same recommendation. The golden rule of "Do unto others as you would have them do unto you" is almost universal. It is a phrase that has done a great deal of good for humankind. But as Dr. Hans Selye has said, "strict adherence to such behavior is incompatible with the laws of biology...egotism is an essential feature of all living beings, and, if we are honest with ourselves, we must admit that none of us actually loves all our fellow men as much as ourselves."

Selye is not advocating the rejection of such a wise-old dictum. Instead he is asking that we enlarge on it. "Earn thy neighbor's love" is his wish. Here we use the term "love" as the feeling of friendship, gratitude, compassion, and respect. To achieve this love, the best and simplest guide is to make yourself as useful as possible. By helping people you earn not only your neighbor's love, you also earn more neighbors. Selye wraps up this concept with a story told by a Nobel Prize laureate.

On a train over the Andes, between Mendoza and Santiago, I sat talking to a Bolivian farmer, and asked him whether he utilized modern fertilizers to increase his harvests. "Oh, no," he said, "that would only create dissatisfaction in my neighbors. I prefer a modest harvest to be on good terms with them." You may say he earned the love of his neighbors by not trying to be too efficient.

Building relationships that are dynamic and alive takes time, and work. If you're really concerned about developing those relationships, you may need to reevaluate your priorities and restructure your daily schedule. Some suggestions follow that you can use to help you give love in those relationships that are a constant source of energy.

Spend Time Regularly with the Ones You Love

This sounds almost too simple to include, and that's the problem. We all know it's essential, but we still let things and people we don't really care about dominate our time. One thing that might help is to think "quality" rather than "quantity." Many people avoid spending time with their loved ones because they think they have to block out an hour or two from their schedules. A quiet five minutes with your spouse before work can really strengthen a marriage. Sharing a lunch break with a close friend can be better than spending an evening with her and the TV set. Regular sharing and interacting with others is a requisite to dynamic relationships.

Evaluate Your Social Obligations

Take a good look at all the club meetings, cocktail parties, service groups, church functions, and civic committees to which you belong. Are they crowding you out of a relationship with someone you care about? I believe everyone should do his or her fair share when it comes to these types of activities, but I also know it can become a burden. You, your family, and your friends are more important than the club's annual fundraiser. If you feel that your relationships are suffering because you are forced to attend too many social obligations, gracefully bow out of the less important ones.

Venture Beyond the Casual Courtesies

When was the last time you discussed your views on immortality with your spouse? Does your best friend even know what you think about nuclear energy? Relationships get a chance to grow when they get past comments about the weather, the job, the family, the World Series. In marriage, you need to see each other as real people, not managers of checkbooks, guardians of the kids' health, or earners of an income. In relationships with others, you need to forget about what they do for a living and pay attention to who they are.

Change the Scenery

Isn't it funny how we fall into patterns? You always chat with your spouse over the dinner table. You meet a friend at a bar. You talk with your minister in his office. No wonder relationships lose their fizz. It's amazing what a little change will do. Take your spouse by the hand and walk to a park bench and talk. Invite your friend over for dinner and let the rest of the family meet him. Take your minister to a play, or if he likes sports, to a football game. Find out how human he is. By changing the scenery, you jar yourself into concentrating more on the individual than on playing expected roles.

Have a Purpose in Mind

I'm all for open-ended conversations and nonstructured get-togethers. However, we often get together with others because it's the thing to do. That's not a very good reason to do anything. Your relationships take on new meaning when you have some sort of goal in mind. Instead of just taking your wife out to eat, why not decide to learn a new dance step together at a local night spot. The next time you invite a couple over, tell them they'll each have to come with a story about something crazy they did in high school. Be adventurous!

Don't Be Afraid to Share Emotions

This is, after all, the foundation upon which a genuine relationship is built. Yet most relationships cover all bases but this one. When your relationship with another person allows you the freedom to uncover those deeper feelings of sorrow, pride, hurt, and fear, you will find that relationship to be a continual source of strength.

Your relationships are, perhaps, your most important possession, so it's important to do everything you can to make them as good as possible. Too many people have turned the whole process of relating to people into a stressful and energy-draining syndrome of ego trips, fear, guilt, worry, and frustration. They are afraid to meet new people and to make new friends. They have become immobilized in that they can't escape the constricting confines of relationships that are counterproductive.

If you're a part of that group, you can begin right now to salvage negative relationships and build new ones. The best place to begin is with yourself. Take a good look at yourself and accept what you see. Take pride in the good things you see and resolve to work on those areas that you feel need improvement. As you begin to do this, it will be easier to accept others for what they are. Finding fault will become a thing of the past. Trying to outdo the other guy or gal will become senseless, since you have nothing to prove. You will become secure in your relationships with others, knowing that their friendships can only add to your life. The peace of mind that accompanies this realization will make your relationships a liberating, exhilarating adventure, and definitely will build energy. Feeling good about yourself and others will fill you with vitality and vigor.

A Three-Phase Plan for Relating to Others

Rate how well you get along with the following people. If a category does not apply to you, leave it blank.

ASSESSING RELATIONSHIPS

RATING: 5–Extremely Well   4–Quite well   3–Average   2–Not very well   1–Quite poorly   0–Terrible

Husband/wife		5	4	3	2	1	0
Mother/father		5	4	3	2	1	0
Your own children		5	4	3	2	1	0
Your brother/sister		5	4	3	2	1	0
In-laws		5	4	3	2	1	0
Your neighbors		5	4	3	2	1	0
Your immediate supervisor at work		5	4	3	2	1	0
Your coworkers		5	4	3	2	1	0
Those whom you supervise		5	4	3	2	1	0
Your minister/priest/rabbi		5	4	3	2	1	0
Your landlord		5	4	3	2	1	0
Your friends		5	4	3	2	1	0

SCORING: Total the numbers you have circled. Then divide by the number of categories you rated. For example, if you rated only five columns, and the total rating was 15, your score would be 3.

1-2   You probably have too many negative relationships. Enter at Phase One.

3-4   Most of your relationships are at least satisfactory, though they could use some improvement. Enter at Phase Two.

5   You enjoy your relationships and value improving them. Enter at Phase Three.

Phase One

Keep a log of your positive and negative relationships for one week. (Follow the example below.) At the end of each day, read and reflect on the events listed in the log. Do it again at the end of the week.

MONDAY

APPROXIMATE TIME	PERSON(S) INVOLVED	FEELINGS PRODUCED	POSSIBLE REASON
6:45 A.M.	Wife	Anger— some resentment	Tired— nervous about job.
8:15 A.M.	District manager	Anger/frustration	His arrogant attitude.
9:30 A.M.	Secretary	Mild anger	She didn't warn me about the district manager.
11:00 A.M.	Jim	Enjoyment	Had a few drinks together. He listened to my story.

When you look back at your log, try to see how (and if) your feelings are caused by the person involved or some other factor. In the example, you would think the subject would have reason to complain about his relationships with his wife, district manager, and secretary and that his only true friend was Jim. Actually, his wife and secretary had nothing to do with his anger. Both may, in fact, be very supportive. The district manager appears to be the real culprit. And once the meeting is over, he could have a few drinks with a chimpanzee and still feel enjoyment. Jim may not be a friend as much as a sounding board.

Examine your positive and negative relationships to see what may contribute to them.

Phase Two

Write down the one person with whom you would most like to see an improvement in your relationship.

EXAMPLE

My wife   _____

List three things about that person that you think contribute to your poor relationship.

Never talks with me.   _____

Spends too much time away.   _____

No longer seems physically attractive.   _____

List three things about yourself that you think contribute to the poor relationship.

Put on a lot of weight.   _____

Never really listen to her.   _____

Have low self-esteem right now.   _____

List three things over which neither of you have much control that seem to negatively affect the relationship.

Financial problems.   _____

Her job is really demanding.   _____

I recently got laid off from my job.   _____

List five things *you* would like to try in an effort to improve the relationship.

Lose some weight.   _____

Take a second honeymoon.   _____

Help around the house more.   _____

Meet her for lunch once a week.   _____

Ask her to help me with my job search.   _____

Select what appears to be the easiest option from the previous list of items and make an effort to try it during the next week.

Repeat this process for two other people. Remember, developing positive relationships takes time. Don't rush through this process. You may need to spend a week or two observing your relationships before you can complete the questions.

NOTE: If any of your relationships seem too difficult to handle yourself, I strongly recommend you consult a professional organization that can offer counseling and advice. Every state has a department of social services with local offices in each county. They may include such services as family counseling, parent training, and various resource people to deal with crises within relationships. Many urban and suburban areas have crisis centers for victims of physical and psychological abuse. Alcoholics Anonymous along with their younger counterpart Al-A-Teen and their family division Al-Anon, are excellent sources if the problem is chemical (alcohol or drugs) related. If you are not sure where to turn for professional help, call your local hospital or check with your religious leader, and ask him or her to refer you to an agency that might help you with your specific problem. Also, a local community college or university can be an excellent source for assistance.

Phase Three

DAILY   Try to speak kindly or offer a word of encouragement to at least one person.

WEEKLY   Hold a family "pow-wow" where the whole purpose is to keep the lines of communication open between all members. Encourage sharing of feelings as well as petty problems that often arise. Spend some time in physical contact, either holding hands in a circle or embracing each other. End the session by singing or reciting an inspiring verse together. Or pray or meditate together.

MONTHLY   Form a small discussion/sharing group. Contact 3 to 5 people with whom you would like to engage in conversation and emotional involvement. During the first few meetings, you may have to initiate conversation by putting thought-provoking questions in a hat and having each member draw one. Forego the usual "party" format of games, drinks, dancing, etc. Use the time to develop strong bonds of genuine friendship.

YEARLY   Try to develop and cultivate one new relationship. Look around. Is there a neighbor, coworker, relative, student, etc., that you would really like to know better? In the past, have you felt a little inhibited about initiating a relationship? Reach out and treat yourself to another exciting adventure. Your goal is to allow the relationship to develop beyond the casual stage and into a close bond of friendship.

▶▶ Section IV: ▶▶

Taking Charge

Your Life Force

Very few people do everything right. If they eat right, maybe they offset the advantages of proper diet by drinking too much. They might enjoy rewarding and productive relationships but be miserably out of shape. Or maybe they're so skinny they are unable to enjoy proper rest and relaxation. Certain negative aspects of these people's lifestyle make you suspect that they would suffer from a debilitating lack of energy. But not so. They have hustle and drive, they're getting a lot from life, they are the eternal optimists, and no obstacle is too big for them. They are storehouses of energy.

What do they have going for them? Any number of things is possible, but I suspect that underlying everything is a powerful life force that results in a healthy self-image. These people like themselves. They aren't necessarily conceited; in fact they may be very humble and kindhearted types, but they've accepted themselves. They have arrived at a basic understanding of who they are, and consequently, life isn't particularly threatening.

I know several people like that. Dr. Ellwood Voller, past president of Spring Arbor College, is one. He admits to being 40 pounds overweight and loves to eat scrumptious meals loaded with a lot of things I've told you to avoid. And he is very sedentary. Presidents of colleges find it difficult to escape being sedentary—long staff and board meetings, thousands of miles in cars and airplanes, and plenty of trips on the biscuit circuit. This guy should be perpetually exhausted, right? Well, the law of averages would suggest it, but this gentleman is different. The thing about Ellwood is, he

179

has the enthusiasm, vigor and energy of a puppy. He laps up love and affection as if it were going out of style. Now, if you're living like that, I'm warning you that the cards are stacked against your having enough energy. But Ellwood is an exception. When he was in his 60's, he retired to manage a gold mine. Later he took to farming and raising Angora goats. Now, at the age of 75, he is on the road across the United States selling programs for a local college. He is having the time of his life. He seems to gain energy as he grows older. Everyone who meets him wants to know how he became so special.

His strong will to live—his life force—is the reason for both his energy and his successful life. Ellwood told me that if he had his life to live over again he wouldn't change a thing. He's been a teacher, a coach (high school and college), a counselor, a farmer, and an insurance salesman. He has done virtually everything. He still works until 1:00-2:00 a.m., bounds out of bed at 6:00 or 7:00 a.m., and is perpetually on the go, flying all around the country. He likes himself, can offer nothing but praise for his wife, enjoys his children, does everything in his power to spoil the grandchildren, and he loves people. Leave it to Ellwood to notice when a friend or neighbor needs help. He will stop what he is doing, take off his coat, pitch in, and probably work 80 percent of the rest of the crew right under the table. No job is too big or small. He has energy galore.

Ellwood hasn't done everything right, yet he has get-up-and-go! Why? He probably is blessed with good genes, energy-wise, and he has done the most important things right. He refuses to believe anything except the best about people and human nature, and he knows he has lived a rewarding and productive life. He has a strong life force. No wonder he has an abundance of energy. If it were possible for humans to reach perfection, Ellwood would be knocking on the door—if only he would eat and exercise properly!

You won't do everything right either. In fact, the chances are good that you, like many Americans, are doing virtually everything wrong. To top it off, you may have a weak ego. You may be convinced that "the force" is not with you. You may feel like a nobody. Disappear, and who would miss you? The political system has become so big that you may have concluded that your vote won't make a difference, your protest won't be heard, your convictions will be trampled. You may have become so much a part of the industrial machine that you've lost your identity. So you try to find yourself and derive your energy from extraneous sources.

Sociologists tell us that this reaction is normal for children. The young child does not clearly distinguish between who he is and what he has. Instead of thinking, "I am," the child says, "I *have*...a mother...a father...a toy truck...a doll." He finds his identity in the things that he possesses. For children this is no problem. The question is, have you outgrown this "I have, therefore I am" thinking?

As the child in you matures, you will gain possession of yourself. Your need to possess external objects will be reduced. Having your own crayons will become less important than just being able to color with any old crayons. You won't need a nicer car every year. Getting there will be all that matters, whether by walking, taking the bus, or being in a car pool.

No longer will you be manipulated by those whose only motive is to make a buck. Never again will you let poor relationships drain your energy. Temporary setbacks won't trip you up or turn you loose on binge eating or drinking sprees. Ultimately you will acquire the life force quotient of the Quakers I grew up with in Pennsylvania. One of my favorite jokes, which exemplifies their humor, energy, and zest for life, goes like this: A Quaker was leaning on his fence watching a new neighbor arrive. After the movers had carted in all sorts of fancy appliances, electronic gadgets, furniture, and costly wall hangings, the Quaker called over, "If you find you're lacking anything, let me know and I'll show you how to live without it."

This gentleman knew who he was and felt totally free of the social pressures that plague most of us. He was doing without negative addictions, labor-saving gadgets, and the constant struggle to balance the checkbook. He saw the humor in life situations, and he had no lack of energy. Why? Because of a lifestyle based on a secure sense of identity—a strong life force.

My friend Ellwood is the same way. He is doing more than just coping with life. He has mastered living. Think about it for a minute. You know people like that too. They may not have much going for them. Not all are that good-looking, their clothing may be slightly outdated, and they may not have particularly amazing talents. Yet they have friends everywhere, always seem to be ahead of the eight ball, and suddenly you realize that even you (who are really quite choosy about who and what you will put up with) really like these individuals yourself and enjoy seeing them. You want the life force they have. You like them because they like themselves.

Fostering a Strong Life Force

In order to acquire the life force they exhibit, begin by liking yourself. Psychologists call this self-love. I touched on this in the last chapter. By self-love I do not mean conceit. You do not go around bragging about yourself, drawing attention to your achievements, thumping your chest, or boasting. Conceited people, just like those who dislike themselves, evaluate themselves on the basis of how others see them. Self-love, on the other hand, is internal acceptance with no need to convince others of your worth. What others think is of no consequence as far as your opinion of yourself is concerned. Naturally, you care about being accepted, being loved. But not to the point that your every action is carefully orchestrated to present a particular image of yourself for others to evaluate.

Maybe you don't like yourself because of the way you perform, whether it's at work, in bed, on the tennis court, or in the kitchen. If so, stop and think about it for a minute. What does performance have to do with self-worth? Absolutely nothing. Recognize that your self-value does not depend upon achievement. Performance implies that you're comparing yourself to some standard outside of yourself. Are you up to par? Don't worry about it. In the game of self-esteem there is no par. Playing the game as well as you can and having an enjoyable time doing it is the only rule. Don't confuse your own self-esteem with anyone else's approval.

There was a popular song in the 1970's that states, "You can't please everyone so you gotta please yourself." While that may strike you as egotistically selfish, there's a lot more truth in that than many like to admit. The first part of that phrase, in fact, is an unalterable truth that you had better reckon with. Regardless of how hard you try, you can't be all things to all people. Politicians consider it a landslide when they get more than 60 percent of the vote. They don't consider the fact that 40 percent of the voters were against them. They can't. They have to go with their strength— their broad base of support—and let the chips fall where they may. For the rest of us the important thing is to be able to please ourselves by becoming who we were meant to be. Some folks will still approve while others will disapprove, but at least you'll approve, and that's one of the secrets to a powerful life force.

This book is not intended to tell you how to love yourself, build self-esteem, and learn to not only tolerate but actually enjoy your fellow humans. That would be downright presumptuous on my part, particularly since there are already dozens of books on this subject in your local bookstore, if not on your own shelves. But these factors have a powerful influence on your life force. As I have shown, a strong life force can be a major source of energy. I recommend that you consider the following in order to enhance your life force.

Know Yourself

Philosophers have been recommending this for centuries. They spend years evaluating themselves and society to determine the extent of self-knowledge and to point out how much better life would be if only each member of the human race knew himself or herself and what he or she was about.

Be Honest with Yourself

"Don't kid yourself" is a common phrase in our society. But in spite of the free advice, a lot of us do try to pull the wool over our own eyes as well as over the eyes of others. There is a fear that recognizing who and what we really are would devastate us. Exactly the opposite is true. Getting honest with yourself is basic to achieving your life force potential.

Have a Strong Sense of Self-worth

All of your feelings about yourself are based on this. Until you come to decide that you have intrinsic value as a human being, and that regardless of what others think or say, you're okay, you will never be able to reach your full energy potential. This is the essence of a powerful life force—a basic liking for yourself that enables you to make a contribution to the world, your society, and your family.

Be Adaptable to Change

There will always be change. Everything else will change. So obviously, you're going to have to learn to adapt.

Accept Others

There are a lot of strange people in the world. Almost none of them are like you—attractive, brilliant, amiable, clever, and mature. Most of them are stupid, boorish, ugly, childish, or uptight. In addition to that, they might be communists, klansmen, revolutionaries, animal rights demonstrators, or snobbish intellectuals. They support politicians you abhor, root for athletic teams that you wish to see badly beaten, and even drive Fords in spite of the fact that you are convinced that no vehicle besides the Chevrolet ought to be allowed on the road.

I'm recommending that you accept these individuals and willingly share the planet with them. Look for their admirable traits. Allow that they have a right, just like yourself, to seek fulfillment. When you've come to love and accept yourself, you'll want the same for everyone else, regardless of their race, ideology, national origin, religion, genetic make-up, personality, or anything else.

Think for Yourself

This isn't as easy as it sounds. Everything you know has been taught to you from someone else, whether through your parents, your schooling, your conversations with friends, your personal studies and book reading, or your exposure to the mass media: radio, television, film, newspapers, and magazines. So how are you supposed to think for yourself?

Like I said, it isn't easy. But it can be done. The best method is to carefully evaluate the things that you believe or know, determine why you think what you do, and then act. Base your life on the things most important to you. Don't let anyone tell you what your priorities are. Listen to them, though, because their input could be valuable to your knowledge and beliefs. By being open minded and thinking clearly you can constantly build a better base for your own ideas, ultimately to reach a high level of maturity and security, something that you will never achieve by allowing others to run your life, doing your thinking for you.

Go Beyond Self

If you do everything for only yourself you are going to be frustrated. Your life will soon feel hollow and empty. The key to high-energy living is to reach out to others, to see how you can help your neighbors, co-workers and friends. Help them repair a fence, raise their child, bake some rolls or share your time when they are hurting. Life is best when you give, rather than take. Show other people you care. That you have an interest in them. This behavior will not only reenergize you, but it will also help make this world a better place in which to live.

Develop Your Sense of Humor

The motto I've adopted is, "He who laughs, last." Laughter is likely to increase your energy as any other concoction or formula known to man. It's a great way to relieve tension, cope with stress, and induce relaxation. When something is really funny, people are known to clutch their sides, gasp uncontrollably, and literally wilt to the floor. But a sense of humor entails more than this. It means seeing the long-range comedy in short-range tragedy and recognizing that when you respond to difficult situations in mature ways and with a sense of humor, any upset can ultimately work to your advantage.

Accept Responsibility

By this I don't mean adopting an inferiority complex or going around like a whipped puppy all the time. What I mean is, that when you do say something you regret, mistreat someone at home, or make a mistake at work, accept responsibility for your error. Don't blame it on someone or something else. And don't stop there. Accepting responsibility entails doing everything in your power to correct the wrong.

Recognize Your Potential

Why is it that two people coming from identical situations so frequently live

184

in totally opposite ways? One becomes highly successful at whatever she chooses to do; the other wallows in self-pity, never seems able to get ahead, constantly complains about her "fate," and lives all of life in emotional, physical, and spiritual misery. The difference is not in what these two individuals have going for them. Externally, everything is the same. However, one sees the possibilities in life situations; the other sees only the problems. A cross-country coach I know wears a T-shirt that says it well, "Every hill is an opportunity." I like that. My friend Ellwood Voller refuses to allow the very word "problem" to be part of his vocabulary. "There is no such thing as a problem," he insists, "only challenges and opportunities." The difficulties in life that he has turned into challenges and opportunities would have destroyed problem-oriented individuals, while these same "problems" have made him highly successful. Whether you become a winner or a loser depends on whether you recognize your potential, and deal aggressively and creatively with whatever life dishes out. You can achieve your biggest dreams, or be the "victim of your circumstances." It's entirely up to you.

Develop a Sense of Purpose or Mission

In the decade of the 60's, college students the world over experimented with drugs, Eastern religions, all sorts of voodoo, and even old-fashioned asceticism in an all-out effort to "find themselves." Few experienced success. The reason why, according to some scholars, is that human beings are like onions. The deeper you dig into yourself, the more layers you peel off and the smaller you become. And what do you discover? Another layer. Finally there is nothing left but a bad aftertaste.

To find yourself you must go beyond yourself. Without external goals, commitments, or a genuine mission, you will find no meaning in life, no purpose for living, no identity. Regardless of your personal beliefs or religious preferences, it is my conviction that a powerful source of energy is faith in a higher being. This is the real source of the life force. Joan of Arc probably didn't do everything I have suggested for maximum personal energy, but she sure had what it took to be an overcomer. Her life force was intense dedication to her church and loyalty to the Pope. Kamikaze pilots willingly gave their lives in honor of their nation, and for their emperor. Martin Luther King Jr. exhibited limitless energy in his battle for justice, and the reason for his war on the status-quo was rooted in his Christian commitment. Egyptian leader Anwar Sadat and Israeli leader Menachem Begin, though in many ways exact opposites, were both men of faith, though one was Moslem, the other Jewish. You can debate which was right, but you can't question their high motivation—their life force.

Whether your life force is exemplified by a strong commitment to yourself, your government, or your God, without a doubt, this is your main source of energy. Your life force is a comprehensive sort of energy that motivates when all else fails.

Getting to Your Goals ▶▶**18**▶▶

By now you realize that you have a great deal of potential energy. The question is, how do you go about getting to your energy goals? When you were a child, no doubt you wished upon a star, as I did, and went to bed at night hoping and dreaming that a fairy would fly through your open window, wave a wand over your head, and make your dreams come true. After all, it worked for Pinocchio. As we grew older, we set aside our childish dreams. Unfortunately, many of us keep on wishing; for our ship to come in, for a new day, for a better lot in life.

Setting Your Goals

To achieve your energy potential, wishing won't do it. You must set goals. When Martin Luther King, Jr., said, "I have a dream," he touched on something that is basic to the nature of all humankind. King took great strides toward fulfilling his goal and never relented, right up to the moment of his tragic death.

You too have a dream. You would like to achieve maximum personal energy. Maybe you refer to it as your "pipe dream," something you never expect to achieve, but something you love to think about anyway. I am going to show you that it is possible for you to make your dream come true. I assure you that this is not another pipe dream. This is no wish upon a star. This is a proven method whereby you can, in a sensible and methodical process, actually fulfill your energy goal.

If you are older than, say, ten years of age, you probably think that your imagination has been destroyed. You no longer believe in Santa Claus or the tooth fairy or even the Easter Bunny. Somehow you have thrown out your own hopes and dreams along with those fantasies. So the first thing you need to do in order to make your energy dream come true is to take a look around in that huge storage tank that is your brain. Find your imagination. You probably left it in the backyard right next to your broken tricycle. Now put that imagination back to work. Let it run wild. Don't be shy. It's the only way to find out those things that you really want. It's the first step toward achieving your energy goals.

Well, what did you discover? Do you want a face fit for the cover of *Mademoiselle?* Or do you want a body that looks like Charles Atlas? Maybe you want to be able to run a marathon, or have the ambition to build your own home, or improve your marriage relationship. It's possible that your most pressing goal right now is to muster the strength to mow the lawn. The point is, we all have a whole range of goals. Some of them are virtually impossible (like building muscles like Charles Atlas), and some of them highly possible. You will achieve then next week, next month, or by next year.

Right now take out a sheet of paper and make a list. Write down every energy goal you can think of. Call it your wish list. (See Table 18-1). What do you want? A 24-inch waist? The pep to dance the night away? To be vigorous and vibrant at age 95? My buddy, Phil Lancaster, a cerebral palsy victim when he was ten years old, had a goal to walk a half-mile with the aid of his rollator. He trained for a whole summer. It took him an hour and 20 minutes but he did it. Why? He had a goal, a dream. His new goal is a mile. His reward—the satisfaction of a job well done and a trip to Disney World.

Put down all of your goals. If your goals are unrealistic because you think you don't have the money, the time, or the smarts (or the energy), don't worry about it. Write them down anyway. Remember, you're planning not for what you are but for what you can become. Put it down even if you don't think you deserve it.

Okay, have you made your list? If you have, you're probably embarrassed. That's okay, you don't need to show it to anyone else. After all, they are your goals, not someone else's. Chances are, they are more realistic goals than you think, because every desire and ambition that you have is probably nothing more than the seed of some undeveloped talent of yours. If you can clearly visualize it and if you genuinely desire to achieve it, then don't suppose that it is not within the realm of possibility. All that you have done so far is to recognize your potential. The only thing that limits your potential is your own self-imposed boundaries; your own doubts. If you dare to use them, you will discover within yourself great creativity, originality, even brilliance. One of the most practical statements ever made is this time-proven affirmation, "Ask and you shall receive, seek and you shall find, knock and it will be opened unto you." But it's up to you to do the asking, the knocking, and the receiving.

Table 18-1. My Maximum Energy Wish List (Goals)

EMOTIONAL ENERGY

1. _____
2. _____
3. _____

PHYSICAL ENERGY

4. _____
5. _____
6. _____

NUTRITIONAL ENERGY

7. _____
8. _____
9. _____

RELATIONAL ENERGY

10. _____
11. _____
12. _____

MENTAL ENERGY

13. _____
14. _____
15. _____

SPIRITUAL ENERGY

16. _____
17. _____
18. _____

Human energy is like money. As you know, you have to spend or invest money to make money. The same is true of burning energy: it's a smart investment. You get back more than you put out. Let's take developing positive relationships, for example. It takes work. Hard work. You have to really try. You may have to go out of your way to do something nice for someone that's close to you. Yet the results are not only emotionally rewarding, they seem to give you a lift that carries you throughout the day. Instead of being immobilized over a negative relationship, you find yourself enthusiastic about your friends. So the first step in achieving your energy goal is to find that last remaining scrap of energy and put it to work.

Warning: It is not likely that you will ever achieve anything worthwhile overnight, whether it be an energy goal or any other type of goal. Everything good takes time. All of life is a growing, changing process. The only thing about life that doesn't change is change itself. I know there are those who say "I can't help the way I am, I was born this way," but I know that isn't true. No one over a day old has stayed the way he or she was born. We are all constantly changing. Even if you are 40 years old, you are a totally different person than when you were 30, for the simple reason that every one of the billions of cells in your body is replaced every seven years. If you haven't changed, grown, or improved in some way it's only because you don't want to.

Maybe you've heard the old joke about how you were born with two ends, one end for sitting and one for thinking. Your success depends on which end you use—heads you win, tails you lose.

You probably have experienced many successes already even if you don't look at them that way. Don't compare your successes with the successes of others. You are a unique individual. The only comparison that you ever need to make is between what you are now and what you can become. The past is past. Don't let it hold you back. Every day is a chance for a new beginning. Take to heart the overworn but not overpracticed cliche, "Today is the first day of the rest of your life."

The odds are that if you made a very long list, then you covered quite a few areas of your life. It might be a good idea to break them down into five or six different lists. What kind of changes can you make in your social life that will improve your energy? Your family life? Is there room for improvement in your religious or spiritual life? What about physically? Is your body in the kind of shape it needs to be in to realize your maximum personal energy?

Maybe you think this energy list idea is an exercise in futility, but it can work. John Goddard made a list of 127 things that he wanted to do in life. He made the list when he was only 15 years old. For him, the list of goals virtually became a blueprint for his life. Some of his goals were rather easily accomplished. For example, he wanted to become an Eagle Scout and he wanted to learn to type 50 words a minute. He also wanted to milk a rattlesnake, read the entire encyclopedia, and execute a parachute jump. While those goals were a little more difficult, he did manage to achieve them. As a matter of fact, by the age of 47 he had accomplished 103 of the items on his list. Some of his goals, such as climbing Mt. Everest, visiting every country in the world, and going to the moon, are nothing short of fantastic; but it wouldn't surprise me if he achieved them.

In my discussions with some very elderly people, I have discovered a very interesting fact. Very seldom do they talk about things they regret having done. Usually their discussion centers around a list of "things I wish I had done." There's an extremely valuable lesson here. Project yourself into the future. You are now 100 years old. What is it that you regret not having done that you could have done except for your lack of energy or courage? Whatever it is, make that your energy goal.

Achieving Your Goals

You've got your energy wish list. Now how will you get to your goals? You need to devise a plan of attack. Take out your wish list and look it over. Set a deadline for achieving each goal. If your goal was to mow the lawn, you can achieve that by, say, Saturday morning. If you are 25 percent body fat and want to get down to 15 percent, it will probably take a year or so of proper nutrition and considerable exercise.

For each goal, set a deadline that you think is realistic. Your deadline is the first step toward establishing a plan of attack. (See Table 18-2.)

Next, you need to break down your goal into a series of steps that must be taken in order to achieve it. For example, before you can mow the lawn you may need to put a new spark plug in your mower, clean the old grass from under it, and be sure that all of the rocks have been removed from your front lawn. Next, you need a full tank of gasoline and perhaps one, maybe two, hours of spare time. And there you have it; success.

The steps toward becoming vigorous and vibrant and jovial by the age 95 can be broken down in a similar fashion. How much exercise will you need each day to avoid a heart attack? How much of what sort of food should you eat? What negative addictions will have to be eliminated in favor of new, creative, positive addictions? Then, set up a realistic plan for making these changes over the next 2, 5, or 20 years.

For greater emotional energy, maybe you need to be more reliable and trustworthy at work. Perhaps you need to develop your skills as a responsible decision-maker. Is there room for improvement in the way you treat your fellow employees? If your goal is to go to the moon, check out what it takes to become an astronaut. Maybe you, like H. G. Wells, will even need to dream up your own spaceship. That may sound a bit absurd, but the point is, any energy goal can be broken down into its necessary ingredients for fulfillment. In other words, each major goal is the result of a series of miniature goals. Start a sensible plan of attack on each bite-sized goal and become your ideal self, perhaps even sooner than you ever expected.

Table 18-2. Wish List Plan of Attack

	ACTIVITY (GOALS)	PRIORITY	SAMPLE ACTIVITY	SAMPLE PRIORITY
EMOTIONAL ENERGY			Stretch for stress reduction 20 minutes each evening.	1
PHYSICAL ENERGY			Be physically fit— score good or better on a physical fitness test. Stop smoking	4 7
NUTRITIONAL ENERGY			Cut 50% of sugar from diet.	5
RELATIONAL ENERGY			Attend concert, play, or movie with friend once weekly.	3
MENTAL ENERGY			Be able to discuss literature, sociology, and philosophy intelligently.	6
SPIRITUAL ENERGY			Become a culturally and spiritually aware Jew.	2

To guarantee success I recommend that you follow this outline: Take each goal from every category of your life and make a detailed plan for achieving it. What are your daily goals that ultimately will wind up achieving your ultimate goal? What can you do on a weekly basis that will help you get there? Finally, what can you do on a monthly or even yearly basis that will push you toward success? For example, maybe your life goal is to have a green house with plants that are the envy of the entire city. Each day you can water and tend to your plants. On a weekly basis you can do some of the more extensive dirty work such as repotting your plants. Once a month you can buy a new plant and add it to your collection. If you did this, in just four years you would have 48 new varieties of plants. If you're not careful, before you know it you'd have to hire a full-time gardener. But your life's goal could be achieved easily and sensibly.

Break down your energy goal the same way. You might decide that your biggest problem is stress, so you need to start your energy plan by dealing with stress, perhaps through 20 minutes of body scanning each morning and night. This mini-goal can be reached by setting aside the right amount of time each day, and doing your best to insure that you spend this time in the way you intended. Once each week write down how successful you've been at reducing stress. At the end of each month sit back, read through what you've written, think back over the month, and evaluate your stress level. If this technique isn't working for you, try stretching or something else. The goal is the important thing, not how you achieve it. As time goes on and you experience success in this top priority goal, move on to your next priority. By the year's end you may be doing pretty well on stress, but you're fed up with having to have a cigarette every 20 minutes, so you ditch those in favor of a new hobby—say, playing the bagpipes. (See Tables 18-3 and 18-4).

One problem you're going to run into next is deciding which goals you want to achieve first. Maybe you wrote down 20 goals on your wish list. If so, it's not likely you can work on all of them simultaneously. So now's the time to go through that list and rearrange each goal according to priorities. (In determining priorities it will help if you go back and reread Chapter 6). Maybe you don't really want to quit smoking as badly as you want to reduce your passion food consumption. List as top priority those goals that have the most value to you. Don't throw out those other goals, just put them in the background for now. It's a matter of doing first things first. And it's very likely that you will be able to achieve many goals at the same time. You can take up jogging to gain energy to get through the day, and discover that you've lost 15 pounds in the process. You can even go jogging with a friend and thereby build a relationship as well as improve your physical energy. In short, knowing your goals and setting up a plan of attack is almost as good as being able to jump on your horse and take off in all directions at once. By establishing priorities you identify the goals that are most important to you and come a long way toward achieving them. It also saves you a lot of trouble, particularly if you are one of those people who has trouble making decisions. Now you can just ask yourself, "Which option will get me closer to my goal?" By lining up your goals in front of you and recognizing what values are most important, you can eliminate a great deal of the difficulty in decision making. You can wipe out some of the stress of life. Perhaps more important, you'll recognize progress when it happens. True, if you don't know where you are going you will be sure to get there. But that's not exactly what I call success.

Table 18-3. Example of Plan of Attack Breakdown

	Now	**Intermediate**	**Long-Range**	**Goal**
Emotional Energy	Stretch before going to bed.	Compare with last week. More flexible, relaxed?	Compare yourself with a friend who doesn't stretch. See progress?	Stretch for stress reduction and relaxation.
Physical Energy	Walk 15 minutes four evenings a week.	Walk/jog 15 minutes four times weekly.	Jog 15-20 minutes four times a week.	Be physically fit and score good or better on fitness test.
Nutritional Energy	Stop putting sugar on cereal.	Cut pop and cola consumption in half, reduce candy intake, Drink fruit juice instead.	No sugar drinks. All fruit juice. No candy except special occasions. Fresh and frozen foods, less canned goods.	Cut 50 percent of sugar from diet.
Relational Energy	Read paper to know what's going on.	Buy tickets, call friends, attend concert or play.	Produce mini-performance in your own living room once a year.	Get "cultured."
Mental Energy	Keep alert for interesting titles.	Visit library or bookstore, choose book, read 2 books monthly.	Return library books, have party and exhibit your brilliance and wit to friends.	Be able to discuss literature, sociology, and philosophy intelligently.
Spiritual Energy	Read scripture 15 minutes daily. Buy study guide?	Attend synagogue.	Consult Rabbi. Discuss progress.	Become a culturally and spiritually aware Jew.

Table 18-4. Plan of Attack Breakdown

	Now	**Intermediate**	**Long-Range**	**Goal and Date to Achieve It**
Emotional Energy				
Physical Energy				
Nutritional Energy				
Relational Energy				
Mental Energy				
Spiritual Energy				

Getting where you want to go requires more than goals. It requires planning. It requires confidence in yourself. You need to know that your goals are both worthy and attainable. It requires establishing daily habits that push you toward your goals. It demands that you shake off that old "I can't do it" attitude. I believe attitudes are based on behavior. Change what you do, and improved attitudes will result. Instead of leaving it up to someone else, you will start thinking in terms of "leave it to me." The energy buck stops with you.

When a Goal Is Achieved

Even if you have always thought of yourself as a failure, by following the outline I have suggested above you are going to begin immediately to enjoy success. You did relax by stretching for 20 minutes last night just as you planned. You have been losing a pound a week for the last two months by burning the extra calories in aerobic activity. That makes you almost 10 pounds lighter. Things are going better in your marriage because you've started treating your spouse the way you wish he or she treated you. Your goals, no matter how small, are being achieved. Your dreams are coming true. You are a success. Now, how are you going to cope with the new you? How do you deal with this new confidence and self-assurance that you've been feeling lately?

The first thing you could do is take the time to enjoy yourself and your achievements. Celebrate! Tell your friends how much you are enjoying your newfound energy as well as the new pattern of living you've adopted. Rejoice in the fact that you are growing and developing into the person that you want to become.

The novelist John Steinbeck said, "It is the nature of man to rise to greatness if greatness is expected of him." When you set out to achieve your goals you are expecting something of yourself. It's almost like a self-fulfilling prophecy. Have you ever noticed how children tend to behave pretty much the way you expect them to? You are the same way. Now that you are expecting an energetic life for yourself, you are accomplishing it, and you are also enjoying life more.

There is the danger that, as you become more and more goal-oriented, rather than enjoying success once you have achieved your goal, you might tend to become like a Buddhist friend of mine who works for a nationally known engineering firm. For the last 2 1/2 years he has been working extremely hard for a promotion. The hoped-for promotion came last month. Is he enjoying it? Evidently not. When I talked to him a short while ago it was almost as though he had forgotten that his current job had ever been a goal. He did not appear to be enjoying it at all. Rather, he already had his eye on a further goal that will take at least 5 years to achieve. His problem is that he has become excessively goal-oriented to the extent that achieving goals no longer brings satisfaction. Don't get caught in that trap. When you reach an energy goal you have been working toward, make the most of it. Enjoy yourself. By doing so it will become possible to make great progress and also to enjoy your present circumstances.

Remember the words of H. G. Wells: "Success is to be measured not by wealth, power, or fame, but by the ratio between what a man is and what he might be."

The Go Power of Positive Addictions

W e're almost there. In the first part of this book we talked about the stressful society we live in and why getting energy can be so tough. Then we evaluated all of the energy options, from rest to relationships, from stretching to strategies for fat-fighting, from yoga to aerobic exercise. You discovered that your life force can make a huge difference in your energy, and then learned that it is possible to reach your maximum personal energy goals.

The chances are good that you don't agree with everything I said, and maybe you're worried that it will be impossible to put into practice the things you do agree with. That's the reason for this final chapter, an explanation of how you make maximum energy a part of your everyday life.

I want to convince you beyond the possibility of doubt that maximum personal energy is yours for the taking. The way to get it is through the "go power" of positive addictions.

We abuse ourselves and rob ourselves of energy by choice—by excesses in our living. We think we're trapped into a nonenergetic life by our jobs, religion, spouse, culture, habits, everything. But we're not. Our problem is that we are living within self-imposed boundaries. We are victims of our own negative addictions.

A negative addiction is anything that takes away your life force—your energy—and gives nothing in return. Negative addictions destroy you in some way, either physically, emotionally, spiritually, or any combination of the above. The symptoms of addictions are numerous: fear, anger, worry, aimlessness, chronic complaining, blaming others for unhappiness, obsession with money, tension, constant struggling without getting anywhere, fighting life, denying feelings. I could go on, but that would belabor the point and it might depress you greatly. These negative addictions, however, can be dropped, and they can be replaced by positive addictions that lift you up by building you physically, mentally, and spiritually, to maximize your personal energy.

Psychologists present strong arguments insisting that fulfillment, pleasure, recognition, a sense of personal worth, loving, and being loved by others are not optional ingredients to your energy. They're requirements. When you get addicted to things that improve your life in any of these ways, you become a junkie—a positive addiction junkie.

Positive addictions provide their "users" with added strength, more confidence, more creativity, better health, more happiness, direction, a sense of well being; in short, everything you need for energy. Such activities include swimming, yoga, cycling, meditation, prayer, stretching, relaxation, response activities, knitting, crocheting, needlepoint, tatting, gardening, writing a personal journal, playing a musical instrument, hiking, weight lifting, cross-country skiing, bicycling, bird watching. One man I know spends an hour every day mulling over a chess set. Unless you're a chess expert he can clean your clock. But he doesn't spend an hour a day staring at the squares and moving the pieces to beat or destroy you. He does it because it calms his nerves. It makes the rest of his life easier to master.

To explain why I believe positive addictions are possible, I need to talk about cause and effect. Take negative addictions for example. A major cause of negative addiction is not merely that people are looking for pleasurable experience by getting high, or drunk, or just getting through the day. They are driven to it by a fear of failure or rejection, a lack of love and acceptance, as a result of peer pressure—any number of reasons. The negative addiction is the means of adapting to their environment, getting along with their acquaintances, as an escape from the pain of poor relationships or a lousy self-image, or handling change. Although the relief is temporary at best, it is something. That is the main motivation: a brief escape and a relief from the pain. The rush of pleasure that often accompanies the negative addiction fix is an extra plus, or is considered so by the user.

Pain, misery, and suffering are for the purpose of telling you something is wrong. At one time leprosy was a much dreaded disease, not because it hurt, but because of the loss of feeling. It has been established that the loss and disappearance of fingers and toes of lepers was often due to injuries and accidents. The lepers never felt a thing.

You need your feelings. You need pain. Your sensitivity to injury has saved you from irreparable damage more times than you can imagine. So why deal with it with a negative addiction? Why do or take something that saps strength and vitality and gives you nothing in return? Why settle for a life completely devoted to an addiction that will only destroy you and those you love? Why not rather deal with that weakness in your life with the go power of a positive addiction?

Life for a positive addict is something else. He is greedy for life. He welcomes adventure, change, the unknown, the future. He sees injury as an opportunity for growth. He isn't particularly concerned about what others think or say about him. He likes himself and wastes little time concerning himself with what he hasn't got. Rather, he revels in his own uniqueness and relaxes inside of his identity. He has the power to be who he is.

You should recognize that what I have described is an accomplished positive addiction junkie, and you can't become one overnight. But you'll get there. The thing about positive addictions is, once you get hooked, they pull you up. You get high. You not only enjoy your addiction, you also gain mental strength that you then use to help yourself accomplish your goals more successfully: you gain more love, more worth, more pleasure, more meaning, more zest for life, more energy. In time you will find yourself well suited to and comfortable in this energetic life you've latched onto.

How do you get a fix on this positive addiction, this "stuff" of life? Begin by deciding what you'd really like to get hooked on; something you can do for somewhere between a half-hour and an hour a day.

Dr. William Glasser, the man who coined the phrase "positive addiction," says that a positive addiction can be anything you choose as long as it fulfills these six criteria:

1. Something noncompetitive that you can devote about an hour a day to.
2. Something not requiring a great deal of mental effort.
3. Something you can do alone.
4. You must believe it has some physical, mental, or spiritual value.
5. Something that you will improve at if you stay with it, but without an attempt on your part to measure your improvement.
6. Something you can do without criticizing yourself.

There are two major categories of positive addiction: the physical, led by active exercisers; and the mental, dominated by meditators and thinkers. Whatever the method, the results are the same: the positively addicted state of mind. This is the "high" that you can expect to get from your addiction. Meditators try to reach this state directly, by purposefully obliterating negative thoughts. Exercisers arrive at it indirectly, realizing that after the first few minutes of activity, they will break through. Most addicts describe this state as extremely pleasurable, relaxing, and feeling very good. It is a state difficult to reach in any way other than through addictive activities. Also, it is something you achieve on your own, not in a group.

Many positive addicts don't even realize their condition. They just know that it feels good, and they don't want to give up their activity. Fortunately, there is no reason to stop. Their positive addiction not only feels good, it also builds strength and enhances life. The mind flows with the body. There is no conflict, no self-critical interference, no competition. You're not trying to prove anything to anyone. You're in your own groove, with no goals, no stopwatch, no careful calculations to measure improvement; just one mind spinning free.

The positive addicts reach this state on a regular basis, at least several times a week. When in the positive addiction state, they experience a rush of pleasure, something they've learned to crave and have come to expect. At the very least, they've acquired a pleasant, relaxing habit.

There are hundreds of potential positive addiction activities, but walking, running, yoga, and meditation are the primary practices in which significant numbers of people report reaching positive addiction. Interestingly, the positive addiction state tends to elude you the more you try directly to achieve it. The most you can do is provide optimal conditions for it to happen. The addiction is passive. It happens completely inside your brain. When the conditions are right, zip, you've got a fix. When you're relaxed, satisfied, and noncritical, it can happen. Accept it, enjoy it, but don't single it out as the only pleasure in life. The key to gaining mental strength through positive addiction is self-acceptance to the point that you are able to leave your brain alone long enough to experience the positive addiction state.

Reaching a positive addiction state takes time, and rarely occurs in less than six months of involvement in a given activity. Some people say it took as long as two years for them. Glasser reports that running is the most strenuous but surest way to achieve positive addiction. The results of his questionnaire printed in *Runner's World* indicated that "about 75 percent of the runners who responded and who had been running regularly for a year, at least six days a week for an hour, are addicted. The two questions, 'Do you suffer if you miss a run?' and 'Do you always enjoy your run?' are both answered with an emphatic 'yes.'" Some runners can't describe their positive addiction experience at all, "which makes sense," says Glasser, "because when our minds are totally spun out there is no tangible experience to describe."

Glasser believes that running creates the optimal condition for positive addiction. His reason?

"It is our most ancient and still most effective survival mechanism. We are descended from those who ran to stay alive, and this need to run is programmed genetically into our brains. When we have gained the endurance to run long distances easily, then a good run reactivates the ancient neural program. As this occurs we reach a state of mental preparedness that leads to a basic feeling of satisfaction that is less self-critical than any other activity that we can do alone."

Personally, I believe the same can be said about walking. Along with the physical benefits of activities like running and walking, people are discovering that their mental energy is enhanced and their ability to concentrate is heightened when they become positively addicted to a healthy activity.

Activities like walking, swimming, cross-country skiing, and jogging result in a great release of tension. It provides a powerful release from depression, anxiety, and other undesirable mental states. It's hard to walk and feel sorry for yourself at the same time. It gives you a sense of well-being. Swimmers who have been swimming for a few months feel a confidence and control over their lives. It is rare to meet a dedicated walker, no matter how busy, who considers quitting. The reason for this? It certainly isn't the quest for good health. There are walkers who regularly put in one to two hours a day, whereas good health can be attained with a mere 20 to 30 minutes of walking a day, three or four times a week. It must be an addiction. Runners *need* their run; walkers, their stroll; readers, their book; and gardeners, their hoe. These are good addictions, and there's nothing wrong with them.

The Flow Experience

A researcher by the name of Dr. Mihaly Csikszentmihalyi, an associate professor of Human Development at the University of Chicago, coined the phrase, "flow experience," another term for feeling high. In the flow experience a person becomes totally absorbed in what he or she is doing. There are no distracting thoughts. A person who plays a very serious game of tennis may be totally absorbed and have total concentration on the project at hand. The rock climber or mountain climber is totally absorbed in the prospect of climbing the mountain and focuses totally on the task at hand. The flow experience is really a proper balance between the skills and the challenge itself. The person is not overwhelmed by the flow experience, but rather seems to be in control of it, and as a result immensely enjoys and successfully completes the task at hand.

This happens many times with exercisers. Athletes talk about the "juice" flowing, or "being in the groove." A swimmer might say he or she has glide. They are totally in sync, having perfect rhythm. A neighbor of mine experiences the same thing while working in his garden. After he gets his second wind and gets beyond the physical part of the activity, the hoeing, weeding, and pruning suddenly becomes a totally creative experience in which he's totally immersed.

There are other people who feel they simply become more energetic as they perform their activity. And that's their high. Not the kind of energy which means they can leap buildings in a single bound, but the kind of stamina that makes them feel they could go on forever, that they are invincible, that they could walk all day or swim across the Gulf of Mexico.

The "high" may simply be a satisfaction of a job well done. A close associate of mine tells me that she has never reached this high and that she really doesn't enjoy exercise per se. But she continues to do her exercises because it makes her feel so good afterwards. "I'm satisfied that I have the discipline to work out 30 to 40 minutes and I feel good about myself and my world." Obviously that statement is symptomatic of increased energy. As soon as you start to feel good or have power, it's bound to increase your energy levels.

Psychiatrist Thaddeus Kostrubala has gone so far as to suggest the possibility that maybe an hour or so of strenuous exercise wipes out the influence of the left cortex, the logical part of the brain, thus allowing temporary dominance of the right cortex, or the artistic and intuitive part of the brain. Sound far out? It's not, really. Many times we simply need an hour or so of repetitive activity to "wipe out" the day's problems and allow us to really dream.

Persistence as the Key

The key to becoming positively addicted to any activity is to do it persistently. It takes considerable self-discipline. After really getting into a positive addiction exercise such as walking you'll discover that it gets gradually easier and easier. The idea of a morning walk seems less threatening. Actually, you've just gotten in shape. You're better. You'll be so encouraged by the results you may even be tempted to maximize the intensity of your training and start walking longer distances.

When you reach this point, watch out. You've reached the negative addiction threshold. A word of caution is necessary here. Like any good thing, positive addictions can become negative, if pushed to extreme limits. The hard-core exercise addict who can't live without the daily run, who experiences withdrawal symptoms when not able or allowed to run, or who runs even when the physician has said "no" has taken positive addiction too far. More than one addict has shown up at the doctor's office on crutches or in a wheelchair as a result of the crippling effects of excessive running.

Runner's World published an article entitled "Jogging About" in which the author, only half-jokingly, proposed that Congress pass legislation requiring the following warning label be placed on running shoes, shorts, and books: "WARNING: The Psychiatrist General has determined that jogging and running are hazardous to mental health and present a grave risk of contracting contagious quasirandomous wanderitis (QW), or 'jogging about.'" The negatively addicted runner ignores pain, may take analgesics before running, and cannot live without the running experience. Job, family, and friends all take a back seat to the all-important run. Clinicians suggest that runners adopt these unconventional priority systems when they run 70 to 100 miles a week. At this point running can become a self-destructive behavior. The key to preventing a negative running addiction is to maintain a perspective that the running program is a means to an end—achievement of positive health, rather than allowing it to become an end in itself.

It is not likely, however, that you will push your positive addiction to that point, particularly if you adopt something other than running for your positive addiction. You may also conclude that the blissful mental thrill or "high" that can come from a positive addiction isn't worth the intense pursuit. Rather, you may be content to take up some relaxing and enjoyable positive addiction to replace a similar negative addiction. For example, if you are in the habit of sitting down in the smoking room after supper and plowing your way through a pack of cigarettes, you may want to acquire a new hobby or skill that requires exercising your lips and diaphragm as well as manipulating the hands. Any activity or hobby can become a positive addiction and can replace any of your old negative addictions. Instead of sapping your energy, positive addictions instill in your body and mind a power for mastery of life that you never considered possible.

The company that tells you to "go for it" doesn't have to tell you what "it" is. That's because we all want "it." You want it. I want it. It's great to have a dynamic, energetic, and vital life. But it doesn't come in a can, a box, or a pill. You can't buy it. No one can give it to you. Yet, a vital energetic life is yours for the doing. Yours, if you are willing to take the risk of being positively addicted, changing your life, and making a commitment to reach your maximum personal energy.

So do it. Master it. Go for it!

►►►►►**Appendix**►►

Appendix A
The Fat-Loss Calorie Counter

Moderate Intensity Activities

Body Weight in Pounds	94-104	105-115	116-126	127-137	138-148	149-159	160-170	171-181	182-192	193+
Calories Burned Per Hour										
Archery	230	245	260	280	295	315	330	345	365	380
Badminton										
Singles-recreational	255	275	295	310	330	350	370	385	405	425
Doubles-recreational	220	235	250	270	285	300	315	335	350	365
Doubles-competitive	335	360	385	410	435	460	485	510	535	560
Baseball										
Pitcher only	285	305	325	350	370	390	410	435	455	475
Catcher only	255	270	290	310	330	350	365	385	405	420
Bicycling-10 mph	300	325	350	370	395	415	440	460	475	505
Calisthenic program-medium	325	350	370	395	420	445	470	490	515	540
Calisthenics-general	220	235	250	270	285	300	315	335	350	365
Canadian XBX-Level 12	220	235	250	270	285	300	315	335	350	365
Canoeing-2 mph	220	235	250	270	285	300	315	335	350	365
Carpentry work-heavy	260	280	300	315	335	355	375	395	415	430
Carrying trays, dishes, etc.- busboy	220	235	250	270	285	300	315	335	350	365
Chopping wood-by hand	330	355	375	400	425	450	475	500	525	550
Dancing										
Aerobic-medium	325	350	370	395	420	445	470	490	515	540
Rumba	220	235	250	270	285	300	315	335	350	365
Square	305	330	350	375	400	420	445	465	480	510
Fencing-recreational	220	235	250	270	285	300	315	335	350	365
Fishing-stream (wading)	220	235	250	270	285	300	315	335	350	365
Gardening-weeding, hoeing, digging, spading	285	305	325	345	365	390	410	430	450	470
Gas station attendant-fix flats and wrecker work	260	280	300	315	335	355	375	395	415	430
Golf										
Twosome, 9 holes in 1 1/2 hours-carrying clubs	275	295	320	340	360	380	400	420	440	460
Twosome, 9 holes in 1 1/2 hours-pulling clubs	245	260	280	295	315	335	350	370	385	405
Gymnastics-light	220	235	250	270	285	300	315	335	350	365
Hiking										
20-pound pack, 2 mph	220	235	250	270	285	300	315	335	350	365
20-pound pack, 3 1/2 mph	280	300	320	340	360	380	400	420	440	465
20-pound pack, 4 mph	330	355	375	400	425	450	475	500	525	550
Horseback riding-trot	300	325	350	370	395	415	440	460	475	505
Hunting (not sitting)	330	355	375	400	425	450	475	500	525	550
Jackhammer (pneumatic tools)	330	355	375	400	425	450	475	500	525	550
Lawn mowing-push	335	360	385	410	435	460	485	510	535	560
Motorcycling-racing	220	235	250	270	285	300	315	335	350	365
Pick and shovel work-continuous	290	315	335	355	380	400	420	445	465	490
Rowing-pleasure, 2 mph	220	235	250	270	285	300	315	335	350	365

Moderate Intensity Activities

BODY WEIGHT IN POUNDS	94-104	105-115	116-126	127-137	138-148	149-159	160-170	171-181	182-192	193+
	CALORIES BURNED PER HOUR									
Rowing machine-easy	220	235	250	270	285	300	315	335	350	365
Sawing-by hand	285	305	325	350	370	390	410	435	455	475
Scuba diving	330	355	375	400	425	450	475	500	525	550
Sex-intercourse (aggressor)	220	235	250	270	285	300	315	335	350	365
Skating-leisure										
Ice	255	275	295	310	330	350	370	385	405	425
Roller	255	275	295	310	330	350	370	385	405	425
Skin diving	330	355	375	400	425	450	475	500	525	550
Sledding	310	335	355	380	405	425	450	470	495	520
Snowshoeing, 2.2 mph	280	300	320	340	360	380	400	420	440	465
Stacking lumber	280	300	320	340	360	380	400	420	440	465
Stationary bicycle (resistance sufficient to get pulse rate to 130)-10 mph	305	330	355	375	400	420	445	465	490	515
Stone masonry	280	300	320	340	360	380	400	420	440	465
Swimming-crawl										
20 yards per minute	220	235	250	270	285	300	315	335	350	365
30 yards per minute	305	330	350	375	400	420	445	465	480	510
Table tennis										
Recreational	220	235	250	270	285	300	315	335	350	365
Vigorous	330	355	375	400	425	450	475	500	525	550
Tennis										
Singles-recreational	310	335	355	380	405	425	450	470	495	520
Doubles-recreational	220	235	250	270	285	300	315	335	350	365
Doubles-competitive	310	335	355	380	405	425	450	470	495	520
Treadmill										
3 mph	220	235	250	270	285	300	315	335	350	365
4 mph	255	270	290	310	330	345	365	385	405	420
Volleyball-recreational	255	275	295	310	330	350	370	385	405	425
Walking										
3 mph	220	235	250	270	285	300	315	335	350	365
3 1/2 mph	230	245	265	280	300	315	330	350	365	385
4 mph	255	270	290	310	330	345	365	385	405	420
4 1/2 mph	330	355	375	400	425	450	475	500	525	550
Upstairs-normal pace	330	355	375	400	425	450	475	500	525	550
Downstairs-normal pace	330	355	375	400	425	450	475	500	525	550
Weeding	220	235	250	270	285	300	315	335	350	365
Weight training (does not include super sets)	220	235	250	270	285	300	315	335	350	365

Moderate-High Intensity Activities

Body Weight in Pounds	94-104	105-115	116-126	127-137	138-148	149-159	160-170	171-181	182-192	193+
Calories Burned Per Hour										
Badminton-singles, competitive (vigorous)	445	480	510	545	575	610	645	675	710	740
Basketball										
Nongame, 1/2 court, etc.	405	435	465	495	525	555	585	615	645	675
Officiating	405	435	465	495	525	555	585	615	645	675
Bench stepping-30 steps per minute, 7 inches	445	480	510	545	575	610	645	675	710	745
Boxing (sparring only)	400	430	460	490	520	550	580	610	640	670
Calisthenic program-high	405	435	465	495	525	555	585	615	645	675
Canadian 5BX-Chart 1A	375	400	430	455	485	510	540	565	595	620
Canadian XBX-Level 24	375	400	430	455	485	510	540	565	595	620
Canoeing-4 mph	450	490	525	560	595	625	660	695	730	765
Dancing-polka	395	425	455	480	510	540	570	600	630	655
Digging	365	390	420	445	475	500	525	555	580	610
Fencing-competitive (vigorous)	445	480	510	545	575	610	645	675	710	745
Football										
Playground-touch	435	470	500	535	565	600	630	665	695	730
Officiating	405	435	465	495	525	555	585	615	645	675
Gymnastics-medium	375	400	430	455	485	510	540	565	595	620
Handball										
Cut-throat	435	470	500	535	565	600	630	665	695	730
4 people	375	400	430	455	485	510	540	565	595	620
Hill climbing	435	470	500	535	565	600	630	665	695	730
Horseback riding-gallop	435	470	500	535	565	600	630	665	695	730
Mountain climbing	435	470	500	535	565	600	630	665	695	730
Orienteering	435	470	500	535	565	600	630	665	695	730
Ropeskipping										
50-60 skips per minute (left foot only)	375	400	430	455	485	510	540	565	595	620
70-80 skips per minute (left foot only)	405	435	465	495	525	555	585	615	645	675
Run in place										
50-60 steps per minute (left foot only)	375	400	430	455	485	510	540	565	595	620
70-80 steps per minute (left foot only)	405	435	465	495	525	555	585	615	645	675
Skating-vigorous										
Ice	455	485	520	555	590	620	655	690	720	755
Roller	455	485	520	555	590	620	655	690	720	755
Skiing-downhill (continuous riding and lifts not included)	435	465	500	530	560	595	625	660	690	720
Snowshoveling-light	445	475	510	545	575	610	645	675	710	745
Soccer	435	470	500	535	565	600	630	665	695	730
Swimming-crawl										
35 yards per minute	395	425	455	480	510	540	570	600	630	655
40 yards per minute	435	470	500	535	565	600	630	665	695	730
Tennis-singles, competitive	435	470	500	535	565	600	630	665	695	730
Volleyball-competitive	435	470	500	535	565	600	630	665	695	730
Walking-5 mph	405	435	465	495	525	555	585	615	645	675
Water skiing	350	375	405	430	455	480	505	535	560	585

High Intensity Activities

Body Weight in Pounds	94-104	105-115	116-126	127-137	138-148	149-159	160-170	171-181	182-192	193+
Calories Burned Per Hour										
Basketball-game (full court, continuous)	545	585	630	670	710	750	790	830	870	910
Bicycling-13 mph	480	515	550	585	620	655	690	725	760	795
Canadian 5BX-Chart 2A	470	505	540	575	610	645	680	715	750	785
Canadian XBX										
Level 36	480	515	550	585	620	655	690	725	760	795
Level 48	575	620	660	705	750	790	835	875	920	960
Dancing-aerobic (high)	480	515	550	585	620	655	690	725	760	795
Gymnastics-hard	520	555	595	635	670	710	750	785	825	865
Handball-2 people	565	610	650	695	735	775	820	860	905	945
Jogging-5.5 mph	480	515	550	585	620	655	690	725	760	795
Judo	575	620	660	705	750	790	835	875	920	960
Karate	575	620	660	705	750	790	835	875	920	960
Martial arts	575	620	660	705	750	790	835	875	920	960
Ropeskipping-90-100 skips per minute (left foot only)	480	515	550	585	620	655	690	725	760	795
Rowing-vigorous, 4 mph	480	515	550	585	620	655	690	725	760	795
Rowing machine-vigorous	480	515	550	585	620	655	690	725	760	795
Run in place-90-100 steps per minute (left foot only)	480	515	550	585	620	655	690	725	760	795
Running										
5.5 mph	480	515	550	585	620	655	690	725	760	795
7.5 mph	510	550	585	625	660	700	735	775	810	850
Skiing-cross country, 5 mph	510	550	585	625	660	700	735	775	810	850
Stationary bicycle (resistance sufficient to get pulse rate to 130)-15 mph	480	515	550	585	620	655	690	725	760	795
Swimming-crawl, 45 yards per minute	500	540	575	615	650	690	725	765	800	835
Trampolining	575	620	660	705	750	790	835	875	920	960
Treadmill-5.5 mph	480	515	550	585	620	655	690	725	760	795
Walking-5.5 mph	480	515	550	585	620	655	690	725	760	795

Very-High Intensity Activities

Body Weight in Pounds	94-104	105-115	116-126	127-137	138-148	149-159	160-170	171-181	182-192	193+
Calories Burned Per Hour										
Bench stepping-30 steps per minute										
12 inches	585	625	670	715	755	800	840	885	930	970
16 inches	810	870	930	990	1050	1100	1170	1230	1290	1350
18 inches	1020	1095	1170	1245	1325	1400	1475	1550	1625	1700
Canadian 5BX										
Charts 3A & 4A	700	755	805	855	910	960	1010	1065	1115	1170
Charts 5A & 6A	705	760	810	865	915	970	1020	1075	1125	1180
Football-tackle	610	660	705	750	795	835	885	930	975	1020
Hockey										
Ice	655	705	755	805	850	900	950	1000	1045	1095
Field	655	705	755	805	850	900	950	1000	1045	1095
Lacrosse	655	705	755	805	850	900	950	1000	1045	1095
Ropeskipping										
110-120 skips per minute (left foot only)	655	705	755	805	850	900	950	1000	1045	1095
130-140 skips per minute (left foot only)	875	940	1005	1070	1135	1200	1265	1330	1395	1460
Run in place										
110-120 steps per minute (left foot only)	655	705	755	805	850	900	950	1000	1045	1095
130-140 steps per minute (left foot only)	875	940	1005	1070	1135	1200	1265	1330	1395	1460
Running										
8 mph	585	625	670	715	755	800	845	885	930	975
8.7 mph	655	705	755	805	850	900	950	1000	1045	1095
11.4 mph	890	955	1025	1090	1155	1220	1285	1355	1420	1485
12.5 mph	1135	1220	1300	1385	1470	1555	1640	1720	4805	1890
Skiing-cross country, 9 mph	730	785	835	890	945	1000	1055	1105	1160	1215
Snowshoveling-heavy	770	825	885	940	995	1055	1110	1170	1225	1280
Sprinting	1780	1915	2045	2180	2310	2440	2575	2705	2840	2970
Stationary bicycle (resistance sufficient to get pulse rate to 130)-20 mph	650	700	745	795	840	885	935	985	1030	1080
Swimming-crawl, 55 yards per minute	610	660	705	750	795	835	885	930	975	1020
Treadmill										
7.2 mph	585	625	670	715	755	800	845	885	930	975
8 mph	655	705	755	805	850	900	950	1000	1045	1095
Walking-upstairs, 2 at a time, rapidly	730	785	835	890	945	1000	1055	1105	1160	1215

Appendix B:
Calorie Content of Food

Food	Amount	Calories
Apple	1 small	100
Apple Cider	3/4 cup	75
Apple Pie	Average piece	400
Applesauce, Canned	1/2 cup	50
Apricots	5 medium	95
Asparagus	12 stalks	25
Avocado	1 small	425
Bacon, Fried	3 strips, crisp	100
Banana	1 medium	100
Barbecued Spareribs	6 average ribs	350
Beans, Baked	1 cup	200
Beans, String	1 cup	25
Beef Bouillon	1 cup	25
Beef, Filet Mignon	Average serving	250
Beef Roast	Average serving	200
Beef, Swiss Steak	1 1/2 ounces	150
Beer	12 ounces	150
Beets	1/2 cup	35
Biscuit, Buttermilk	2 small or 1 large	110
Blueberries, Fresh	1 cup	100
Blueberry Pie	Average piece	375
Bologna	2 ounces	125
Bourbon	1 shot	100
Brandy	1 shot	75
Bread, Corn	2-inch square	200
Bread, White	1 slice	65
Bread, Whole Wheat	1 slice	65
Broccoli	1 cup	45
Brownies	2-inch square	150
Butter	Average pat	40
Buttermilk	1 cup	85
Cabbage, Green, Boiled	1 cup	40
Cake, Chocolate	Average serving	250
Cake, Sponge	Average piece	125
Cantaloupe	1/2 medium	50
Carbonated Beverages	1 average	75
Carrots, Raw	1 medium	25
Catsup	1 tablespoon	25
Champagne, Domestic	1 glass	85
Cheese, American	1 slice	100
Cheesecake	Average slice	350
Cheese, cheddar	1 1/2 ounces	150
Cherry Pie	Average piece	350
Chewing Gum	1 stick	6
Chicken, Barbecued	Average serving	200
Chicken, Fried	Average serving	325
Chicken Roasted	Average serving	250
Chicken Salad	Average serving	225
Chili Con Carne	1/2 cup	250

Food	Amount	Calories
Chocolate Bar	Average	250
Chocolate Chip Cookies	3 small	65
Chocolate Milk	1 cup	225
Chop Suey, Beef	1/2 cup	275
Cinnamon Toast	1 slice	200
Clam Chowder, New England	Average portion	225
Coffee, Black	1 cup	0
Coffee, with Cream	1 tablespoon cream	30
Coffee with Sugar	1 teaspoon sugar	18
Cola	6 ounces	75
Cole Slaw	6 ounces	20
Corn Flakes	1 ounce or 1 cup	100
Corn Fresh Frozen	1 cup	140
Corn Oil	1 cup	120
Corned Beef Hash	1/2 cup	150
Cottage Cheese	1 cup	215
Crackers, Saltines	6 2-inch squares	100
Cream Cheese	1 tablespoon	50
Cucumber	1 8-inch	20
Cupcake	1 small	100
Custard	1/2 cup	125
Daiquiri	1 cocktail	125
Doughnut	Average	150
Dressing, Thousand Island	1 tablespoon	100
Egg	1 average	75
Egg, Fried	1 average	100
English Muffin	1 average	150
Fish, Tuna, Canned in Oil	1/2 cup	250
Frankfurter	1	125
French Onion Soup with Croutons	1 cup	150
Fruit cocktail, Canned	Average serving	100
Fruit Jam	1 tablespoon	50
Gin	2 ounces	150
Goulash, Hungarian	Average serving	350
Grapefruit	1/2 small	50
Haddock, Baked	Average serving	180
Ham, Baked	Average slice	350
Ham, Smoked	Average serving	450
Hamburger, Broiled	2-ounce patty	200
Hamburger, Fried	2-ounce patty	225
Honey	1 tablespoon	65
Hot Fudge Sundae	Average serving	400
Ice Cream, All Flavors	Average scoop	150
Lamb Chop, Broiled	1-inch thick	250
Lamb Roast	Average serving	200
Lemonade	1 cup	100
Lentil Soup	1 cup	300
Liver, Beef	Average serving	150
Lox	2 ounces	200
Macaroni and Cheese	1/2 cup	225
Malted Milk, with Ice Cream	1	400
Manhattan	1 cocktail	175
Margarine	1 tablespoon	100
Martini	1 cocktail	125
Mayonnaise	1 tablespoon	100
Meat Loaf	Average serving	225

Food	Amount	Calories
Milk, Whole	3/4 cup	125
Muffin, Blueberry	1 average	110
Mushroom Pizza	1/6 12-inch diameter	200
Mushroom Soup, Creamed	1 cup	200
Nectarine	1 medium	50
Noodle Soap	1 cup	125
Oatmeal, Cooked	1/2 cup	75
Omelet	2 eggs, 1 teaspoon butter	185
Omelet, Western	Average	325
Orange	1 medium	75
Orange Juice	6 ounces	75
Oyster Stew with Milk	1 cup	200
Oysters, on the Half Shell	6 medium	50
Pancakes, with 2 Teaspoons Butter, 2 Tablespoons Syrup	3 (4-inch, diameter)	470
Peach, Fresh	1 medium	50
Peaches, Canned in Syrup	2 halves	125
Peanut Butter	1 tablespoon	100
Peanuts	10	100
Pineapple, Canned	1 slice	75
Pineapple Upside-Down Cake	Average piece	250
Popcorn, Plain	1 cup	50
Pork Chop, Broiled	1 medium	225
Pork Chop, Fried	1 medium	250
Pork Roast	Average serving	200
Potato, Baked	1 medium	125
Potato, Boiled	1 medium	150
Potato Chips	1/2 cup	100
Potato, French Fried	6 average	100
Potato, Hashed Brown	1 medium	225
Potato, Mashed with 1 Teaspoon Butter and 2 Tablespoons Milk	1 medium	180
Pound Cake	Average slice	125
Pretzels	6 average	100
Pumpkin Pie	Average piece	325
Raisins, Seeded	1/2 cup	225
Red wine	1 glass	75
Rice, Boiled, White	3/4 cup	100
Roll, Plain	1 small	75
Rum, Bacardi	1 1/2 ounces	100
Salmon, Baked	1 serving	250
Sardines, Canned	4	100
Sausage, Pork	2 3-inch links	150
Scotch	1 shot	100
Sherbet, Fruit-Flavored	Average scoop	100
Shortcake, Strawberry	Average serving	350
Shrimp	10 average	100
Skim Milk	1 cup	85
Soup, Bean	1 cup	225
Soup, Chicken Noodle	1 cup	125
Soup, Mushroom, Creamed	1 cup	200
Soup, Tomato	1 cup	100
Soup, Vegetable	1 cup	100
Spaghetti with Meat Sauce	4 ounces	275
Spinach	1/2 cup	25
Squash, Winter, Baked, Mashed	8 ounces	100

Food	Amount	Calories
Stew, Beef	1 cup	250
Strawberries, Fresh	1 cup	50
Stroganoff, Beef	Average serving	350
Sugar, Granulated	1 teaspoon	18
Sweet Potato, Canned	1 cup	235
Sweet Roll	Average	125
Tomato, Fresh	1 medium	25
Tomato Juice	1 cup	50
Turkey	Average serving	175
Veal Cutlet, Broiled	Average serving	125
Vodka	1 ounce	125
Waffle	1	225
White Wine	1 glass	135
Yogurt	1 cup	165

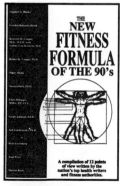